CM0I284670

'According to fashionable "decolonising" theory, European colonists hoisted an alien culture onto unwilling native peoples. Reflecting on his own particular experience in Malaŵi, Alexander Chula tells a less predictable, more fascinating, and far more plausible story of cultural give-and-take. His astute and thoughtful observations of an African microcosm contain important lessons for the larger discussion of the impact of Western colonialism. There is wisdom here, elegantly expressed.'

NIGEL BIGGAR

'*Goodbye, Dr Banda* is one of those rare books that are hard to classify, but are all the more delightful for that very reason. It is a highly unusual personal memoir, but it is also a sympathetic and perceptive portrait of a country and its past. It is a quite superb book that will linger with the reader for a long time after it is read.'

ALEXANDER McCALL SMITH

'This is an impressively researched, beautifully written book. I loved the empathy Chula brings to Malaŵi's myths, our past and our present. The history of missionaries like Robert Laws and Chauncy Maples showed his thoroughness in research. This is a book to read and enjoy.'

FELIX MNTHALI

'A rewarding, delightful and personal examination of Dr Banda's struggle to reconcile his indigenous Chewa culture with the culture of the Greek and Latin Classics. Radical, deep and surprising, with gentle but trenchant observations on African versus Western cultural dynamics, Chula writes with first-hand knowledge of Greek myths and Nyau traditions.'

JOHN LWANDA

'A riveting – and cautionary – tale of a clash of cultures, as seen through the eyes of a young classicist turned medical doctor, who discovers that Ancient Greek legend and the rituals of the Chewa people have much in common. Brilliantly observed and packed with insights, the result is an African classic.'
MICHAEL HOLMAN

'I have read this with great enjoyment. Learning about the tradition of Classics in Malaŵi since Banda is fascinating, and the author's personal experiences as a teacher at Kamuzu Academy – and at Oxford prior to that – are vivid, memorable, and described with directness and elegance.'
ARMAND D'ANGOUR

'Reading Alexander Chula's travelogue, I kept imagining I was soaking in the prose of my travel-writing hero, Bruce Chatwin. Absolutely engaging from beginning to end, *Goodbye, Dr Banda* is very likely to position Chula as a leading literary voice in years to come. I recommend this work for the way it informs, its cultural insights, and for its keenly observed detail.'
TAHIR SHAH,
Author of *Time* magazine bestseller
The Caliph's House: A Year in Casablanca

'Timely, erudite, and a fascinating insight into the complex diversity that is the real modern Africa.'
ROBERT TWIGGER,
Bestselling author of *Red Nile*

GOODBYE, DR BANDA

LESSONS FOR THE WEST FROM A SMALL AFRICAN COUNTRY

ALEXANDER CHULA

Polygon

First published in hardback in Great Britain in 2023
by Polygon, an imprint of Birlinn Ltd

Birlinn Ltd
West Newington House
10 Newington Road
Edinburgh
EH9 1QS

9 8 7 6 5 4 3 2 1

www.polygonbooks.co.uk

Copyright © Alexander Chula, 2023

The right of Alexander Chula to be identified as
the author of this work has been asserted in
accordance with the Copyright, Designs
and Patents Act 1988.

All rights reserved. No part of this publication may be
reproduced, stored, or transmitted in any form, or by
any means electronic, mechanical or photocopying,
recording or otherwise, without the express written
permission of the publisher.

ISBN 978 1 84697 627 8
EBOOK ISBN 978 1 78885 579 2

British Library Cataloguing-in-Publication Data
A catalogue record for this book is available on
request from the British Library.

Typeset in Sabon LT Pro by The Foundry, Edinburgh
Printed and bound by Bell & Bain, Glasgow

To RLH

qui haec mihi monstravit

CONTENTS

Preface   ix

PART ONE: *ET IN MALAŴI EGO*

I	DR BANDA & ME	3
II	THE ETON OF AFRICA	10
III	ARRIVAL	13
IV	THE GREAT TRADITION	19
V	RARE BIRDS	25
VI	THE VILLAGE	34
VII	YOUR PROTOTYPE	41
VIII	CULTURE WARS	45
IX	*GRADUS AD PARNASSUM*	51
X	THE COMMUNICATION OF THE DEAD	56
XI	THE GREAT DANCE	60
XII	DEATH & TRANSFIGURATION	70

PART TWO: NGWAZI

XIII	THE WANDERER	79
XIV	THE GREAT DICTATOR	86
XV	PORTRAIT OF A TYRANT	93
XVI	THE DIALECT OF THE TRIBE	99
XVII	*DE RADICULIS*	106

PART THREE: ONLY CONNECT

XVIII	IN WESTMINSTER ABBEY	113
XIX	*VITAÏ LAMPADA*	118
XX	EVEN UNTO DEATH	124
XXI	INTERLUDE IN ZANZIBAR	130
XXII	*IN MEMORIAM*	135
XXIII	LIVINGSTONIA	141
XXIV	ANCIENT & MODERN	151
XXV	*DEA EX MACHINA*	158
XXVI	PALACES IN THE JUNGLE	167
XXVII	IMPERIAL FOLLY	180
XXVIII	CORNSTALK & LEAF	191
XXIX	ON RUINS	201
XXX	THE USES OF LITERACY	207

PART FOUR: THE NEED FOR ROOTS

XXXI	MODERN TIMES	221
XXXII	SPEECH DAYS	228
XXXIII	THINGS FALL APART	233
XXXIV	THE FORCES OF ENTROPY	243
XXXV	THE AGONY IN THE GARDEN	250
XXXVI	*LUX IN TENEBRIS*	255
XXXVII	LAND OF FIRE	262
XXXVIII	SIGNIFICANT SOIL	270
XXXIX	OLD FIELDS, NEW CORN	277
XL	APOCOLOCYNTOSIS	285

Epilogue   291
Acknowledgements   305

PREFACE

You may never have been, may never go, may never even have heard of the place – but Malaŵi will repay your attention. It is one of the smallest, poorest countries in Africa, often overlooked; but its relationship with us in the West has been extraordinary. A meeting of worlds took place here, between one of the continent's most fascinating indigenous cultures and the best and worst of our own. The story of this is complicated but exhilarating, by turns edifying and deeply uncomfortable. But we would do well to examine it: Malaŵi presents urgent lessons which resonate piercingly in our vexed age of culture wars and identity crisis.

How should we engage with peoples and societies profoundly unlike our own? Westerners wander the earth compulsively, foreign travel assuming an almost existential importance in our lives. Wherever we go, we want to reach out, want to connect. But besides reading the 'history and culture' pages at the back of the *Lonely Planet*, we are often unsure of how to do this – certainly that was my own feeling when I first arrived in Malaŵi. When globe-trotting was suspended by the pandemic, it seemed to me a good occasion to pause and reflect on this.

This book advances no programme or prescription for cultural exchange; rather it observes in Malaŵi a near perfect case study: from Livingstone and the early missionaries, through British colonialists, to today's tourists, expatriates, aid workers and even Madonna, the country has experienced the full gamut of Westerners trying to get to grips with an enthrallingly alien culture. The shared context urges us to weigh these approaches against each other, and against our own. But if the purpose of travel is also to learn something about ourselves, then Malaŵi answers this need too: the country forms a strange, luminous backdrop, against which Westerners appear starkly. Who we are, what we stand for, what we bring to others, for good and ill – all are more perceptible here.

These subjects are approached obliquely, through a mix of history, travelogue, biography and memoir, as I describe the land, its people, and my unlikely presence among them. I first came as a teacher of Latin and Greek, soon after I had completed a Classics degree at Oxford. When I left, it was to study medicine in London, but by then I had grown attached to Malaŵi, so I returned whenever I could. At length I qualified as a doctor and was lucky to be able to go back as a clinical volunteer and experience the country very differently. My impressions – some brief, some extended – were therefore varied and collected over several years.

I came to fixate on how closely interwoven Malaŵi's story is with our own in Britain. It encompasses slavery, imperialism and the struggle for independence, as well as much more recent events. Throughout all this, there has grown a sympathy between Malaŵian and European cultures which runs far deeper than the politics. Embodying this is Dr Banda – Hastings Kamuzu Banda – who lived almost the full hundred years of the twentieth century: a peasant-scholar who became a doctor, a rebel turned reactionary, a champion of African independence who aged into a brutal, senile dictator.

Banda ruled Malaŵi for thirty years until 1994. He was variously monstrous and magnificent, exalted and absurd. My interest in him was stirred by his unusual preoccupations: with culture, identity, belonging. He left home as a boy and wandered to South Africa, America,

Britain. He eagerly adopted the ways of others, but always felt the exile's uprootedness and urge to reconnect. He was infatuated with both Africa and the West, but truly at home in neither. This discord inspired an idiosyncratic vision of how the best of both might be brought together, preserved, and celebrated.

The most flamboyant expression of this was a project to advance his country's development through the study of Greco-Roman civilisation. In the 1980s, he established 'the Eton of Africa', an academy in the Malaŵian bush intended specifically to promote classical education. This institution – or rather its bizarre afterlife – was my introduction to the country. But it also posed the challenge which first impelled me to write this book. I knew from my own student days that Classics had lost its prestige in the West. More and more, the legacy of Greece and Rome was to be forgotten, repudiated, 'decolonised'. What was I to make of such extravagant homage paid to it in Africa? Banda's vision was eccentric and deeply flawed, but, in its problems and paradoxes, it illuminates many of our contemporary uncertainties, especially as we falter towards the ideals of multiculturalism.

As I write, Trafalgar Square's Fourth Plinth has just been adorned with two surprising new statues: of Malaŵian anti-colonial rebel John Chilembwe and an English missionary friend of his. The decision to erect these – in the wake of Black Lives Matter and the toppling of Edward Colston's statue – suggests to me that others also recognise the relevance of Malaŵi's history to contemporary Western concerns. As we shall see, however, the story evoked by the statues is not as straightforward as their sponsors had in mind. Like so much else in Malaŵian history, it is ambiguous, and cuts to the core of the current tense debate about Britain's imperial past.

Trigger warnings are due, although this book perhaps requires more than I can enumerate. Banda was a hero in the struggle for racial equality and against colonialism, but he was also an unashamed elitist, a black man who – in today's parlance – was 'on the side of the patriarchy'. As such, he might have been invented to discomfit modern sensibilities.

There is then the broader historical context of the West's record in Africa, past and present. On this subject, a number of orthodox narratives have come to prevail, but the Malaŵian example does not always reinforce them. In fact, it is frequently subversive.

Lastly, the borrowing and refashioning of others' heritage is pursued with abandon by many characters in this book, most notably by Dr Banda. Our own society has made of this a grave taboo, in fearfulness of being charged with cultural appropriation. But a more equivocal response seems warranted in Malaŵi. If there has been appropriation here, it has not always traduced or diminished. It may even have revitalised and enriched.

Malaŵi is of course materially poor and undeveloped, so it is impossible to skirt over many sad realities of its daily life. My object is never to denigrate; on the contrary, I write primarily in admiration, especially at so much hardship overcome. For despite its poverty, Malaŵian society strikes me as fundamentally healthy. Its peoples are almost quintessentially rooted in time and place, bound by a rich history to their land and each other. Perhaps it is because of this, above all, that the disconnect with our own unsettled culture is felt most strongly. It was long upheld that Malaŵians could only develop with help and guidance from the West. Well, that is for them to decide. But we might now try to invert this way of thinking: today it is the West that should take lessons from a small African country.

PART ONE
ET IN MALAŴI EGO

I

DR BANDA & ME

I had long been aware of the abandoned palace on the hill. It was pointed out to me soon after my arrival in the country, and I observed it from afar with curiosity whenever I drove past. Now at last I was taking the rough road behind the bustling little town that sat beneath, up through the forest to the frayed perimeter fence. It had been arranged for me to catalogue the palace library (whatever was left of it), but I sensed in advance that there might be more to my visit than this. Part of me wondered if I might even find treasure – but I was really looking for something that would shed light on my own perplexing presence in Malaŵi.

My background was suburban, middle class, raised in the West, half English, half Oriental. I grew up amid the unchallenging cosmopolitanism of south London. I was fresh out of Oxford, optimistically equipped for the world with an undergraduate Classics degree. My friends were all knuckling down to serious office jobs back in Britain, so what on earth was I doing in a tiny, impoverished, land-locked country 7,000 miles away? Notionally I was there to teach Latin and Greek – but this answer only prompted further questions.

The approach to the palace was steep, and the views grew wide with the ascent: vast, empty plains to the east; endless dense forest to the west, both unbroken to distant horizons. Minutes before I had been amid noise and squalor, the heat and the dust, assailed by every stereotype of small-town African life: ragged children, bleating livestock, a frenzied market, monstrous trucks. Now, up on the hillside, it was cool, still, quiet. And I remember the smell: the faint, sweet aroma of the surrounding bush, mingled with that of tarmac grown warm in the tropical sun.

The road snaked up to a rusty steel gate that was creaked open by an elderly caretaker. He appeared to be living alone in an adjacent shack, and the place was otherwise deserted. Formal gardens were turning to scrub. Dead leaves choked dried-out fountains. A sapling thrust through a crack in the disused helipad.

I pulled up before the main house, a mass of peeling white stucco, fallen red roof tiles and colonnades entangled by creepers. It had been stripped bare, but a robust, concrete pavilion was set apart from the rest and appeared to be intact. Baboons scattered from the forecourt as I approached. Once inside, the classicist in me gasped with delight: there were dusty books from ceiling to floor. Luxury commingled with decay, like Miss Havisham's house re-imagined in Africa: lion and leopard skins sprawled under foot, tattered by moths; the silk wallpaper was nibbled by termites; cobwebs spanned crystal chandeliers. I set to work on the collection, heaping books and cataloguing them at a large Louis Farouk desk, taking care not to antagonise the wild bees nesting in a corner behind me.

I found an adjoining strong-room, the thick steel door of which had been left ajar. There was no power, so I had to rummage by torchlight: it was all a jumble of packing crates and filing cabinets overflowing with loose papers and bric-à-brac. Only on my final sweep did I notice a small oak casket bound with brass and leather, hidden under a pile of battered oil portraits of Mugabe, Gaddafi, Nyerere. It was unlocked. I took it out into the sunlight and opened it to discover a 1584 edition of Julius Caesar's *Gallic Wars*, printed in Venice by Aldus Manutius, the most celebrated press of the Renaissance. The front page bore a stamp: *EX LIBRIS H. KAMUZU BANDA.*

Dr Hastings Kamuzu Banda. The Ngwazi or 'Conqueror'. And, variously: His Excellency, the Life President of the Republic of Malaŵi, Destroyer of the Federation of Rhodesia and Nyasaland, Father and Founder of the Malaŵi Nation, Messiah, Saviour, Lion of Africa, Doctor of Medicine, Fellow of the Royal Societies of Surgeons & Physicians (Edinburgh), Bachelor of Arts (Indiana), Bachelor of Medicine & Surgery (Tennessee), LRCP, LRFP&S, PHB, Hon. DSc, Hon. LLD (Massachusetts), Hon. LLD (Malaŵi), Hon. LLD (Wilberforce), Hon. LLD (Indiana) and so on.

Even by the Rococo standards of post-colonial Africa, Banda was one of the most astonishing leaders the continent has ever witnessed. He was born just a few miles from the palace, on an uncertain date in the late 1890s. His family were peasants, living in what was then British Central Africa, later known as Nyasaland. Malaŵi was the name Banda chose for the country at independence in 1964.

He had been the first of his family to go to school and was taught by missionaries who came to his village. As a teenager, he walked a thousand miles to South Africa and found work in the mines. He was intelligent and lucky: after several years, he was awarded sponsorship to go to America, where he spent a decade studying Classics, history, literature, anthropology and – finally – medicine. On qualifying, he moved to Edinburgh and later London, where he worked for fifteen years.

As a suburban family doctor in Harlesden, he earned the adoration of his patients, moved in sophisticated circles, joined the Fabian Society, entered the Freemasons, had an affair with a married Englishwoman, canvassed for Atlee's Labour party in the 1945 election and intrigued with African exiles conspiring against imperialism. Never once during this period did he return home.

Malaŵi was part of the 'great interior' of Africa, 'opened up' by Livingstone, then absorbed into the British Empire in 1891. By the 1950s, however, when Banda might otherwise have been contemplating retirement from medicine, independence was in the air. From his semi-detached house in north London, he coordinated a network of anti-colonialist agents who worked to promote his reputation back at home. When he returned for the first time, in 1958, he was welcomed rapturously. The outgoing British administration initially imprisoned him but realised after a year that he was the most popular and best qualified man to take over power. In 1964 he led Malaŵi to independence, won the country's first elections, and then ruled as 'President for Life' for the next thirty years.

His supporters continue to protest the designation 'dictator', but it is difficult to resist. He dispensed with democracy early on and thereafter ruled with authoritarian vigour: 'Everything I say is law – literally law,' he proclaimed. His regime operated by one-party rule and rubber-stamp parliament. There was judicial murder and extra-judicial assassination, defenestration and defalcation; there were cabals, cabinet crises and cult of personality, private extravagance, paramilitary enforcement of petty regulation and parcel bombs posted to overseas dissidents. However, almost until the end of his rule, Banda remained popular. He kept Malaŵi stable, orderly, and out of local conflict – utopian conditions by the standards of the region at that time. Within the limitations of such an undeveloped country, Malaŵi prospered, for a while.

But when I arrived in 2009, Banda was twelve years dead and his achievements lay in ruins. I stood in the empty palace, contemplating the desolation. And what of the mysterious book in my hand? It seemed as out of place as I was. How had a priceless, antique edition of the most famous work of Roman history ended up on a remote mountain in the middle of Africa?

Of course it was Banda's. Like me, he was obsessed with Classics – the study of the Greco-Roman world, its languages, literature, history, culture. His interest began during his early education in America, before he studied medicine. It remained with him all his life and, when he was president, became more and more important to him. Knowledge of the ancient world, he convinced himself, held the key to his country's advancement. And so in 1981 he opened Kamuzu Academy, a boarding school founded specifically so that the nation's ablest children, however poor, might study Latin and Greek.

The 'classical education' emerged in Europe during the Renaissance and came to occupy a central place in the cultural landscape of the West. In nineteenth-century Britain, it was felt to supply the mental equipment that qualified you for government, at home and in the Empire. Banda first encountered its influence in the colonial administrators, missionaries and settlers whom he met in his boyhood.

By the second half of the twentieth century, however, Classics had become an embarrassment. The subject underpinned a historical narrative that lay in tatters after the barbarism of two world wars. The radical politics of the 1960s condemned it as the paradigm of blinkered Eurocentricism, and it began to fade from the school curriculum. But for Banda, Classics still stood for civilisation. Greek and Latin granted access to the wisdom with which the West had flourished: why should it not do the same for Africa? In *The Republic*, Plato envisioned a class of philosopher guardians trained from youth to rule with justice and far-sightedness. The alumni of Kamuzu Academy would assume this mantle and ensure their nation's future.

But the experiment miscarried, and it was only thanks to the strange twilight of Kamuzu Academy that I ended up working there. An attenuated Classics department just about endured into the new millennium, and I learnt that a vacancy had arisen shortly after completing my first degree. I wanted to go to Africa, and it was probably the only job on the entire continent that I was actually qualified to do.

I began to discover odd, sometimes uncomfortable, affinities with Banda. Before I applied to teach at his school, I was already planning the same move from the arts to medicine that he had made in his youth. When I returned to Britain, it was to re-train as a doctor, yet my enthusiasm for Classics stayed with me, as it had with him.

Banda was torn between his African and European identities. Infatuated with both but at home in neither, he spent his life precariously balancing the two. When he returned to Malaŵi after a separation of over forty years, he tried strenuously to recover and reconnect with his own culture while simultaneously promoting the 'high culture' of Europe. I suspect he often felt as much a stranger in Africa as he had while living in the West, everywhere conscious of a rootedness in others that was absent in himself.

I had no connection with Africa before moving to Malaŵi. My father is from Thailand, my mother from England. But like Banda, I've always felt something of a stranger in the two societies where I might claim membership – never unwelcome or ill at ease, just aware of my own difference. Growing up in London, multiculturalism was my norm, but it left me unsatisfied, and I doubted if I could ever properly get to grips with either my Thai or English heritage. But in the classical world there seemed to glimmer an ideal, universal culture that transcended – without negating – contemporary national differences. Clasping Banda's prized edition of Caesar, I surveyed the immense view and wondered if he had felt something similar.

11

THE ETON OF AFRICA

'Latin is not being taught anywhere in the country!' fulminated Banda throughout the 1970s. 'To me, education based on no Latin is a house built on stilts.'

A retired engineer explained to me how the site for Kamuzu Academy had been chosen. Banda wanted the school located beside the very *kachere* tree under which, as a peasant boy, he had received his first lessons at the start of the century. He led a team of surveyors, engineers, and men armed with panga knives into the forest; after three days of grubbing about, the tree was identified and work could begin.

Even promotional material for the school had to admit that its site was remote: somewhere in the country's sparse Central Region, between two immense national parks. Here, a vast tract was cleared, a road constructed, foundations laid. Then dormitories and classrooms, cloisters and laboratories began to rise above the flat horizon. A clock tower, then the tallest structure in the country, was reflected in an artificial lake graced by ornamental fowl and gigantic monitor lizards. The water was pumped several miles from a specially dug reservoir, which irrigated acres of lawns, gardens, golf course, grain and livestock farms. The latter supplied the kitchens, where the produce was transformed into authentic British school meals. At the centre of the whole complex stood a library styled after that of Congress in Washington, DC and equipped with a multi-volume English dictionary donated by Ronald Reagan. A central thoroughfare, called the Appian Way, passed from the Great Hall through hanging gardens beside a Greek theatre. The academy was designed, above all, to produce classicists.

At the opening ceremony, Banda emerged from a helicopter in his signature three-piece suit, Homburg hat and sunglasses. He then knelt to drink at a well remembered from his boyhood before being cheered to a podium by ululating praise singers and warriors brandishing spears and knobkerries. He returned their salute with a cane in one hand, a fly-whisk in the other, before declaring: 'Anyone who does not want to study Latin and Greek has no place at Kamuzu Academy!'

All pupils were required to take these subjects to A level. They were drawn from the best-performing candidates in each district of the country, regardless of social status. Most were poor, and many had never before worn shoes or eaten with a knife and fork. Now they had full scholarships, ties, blazers and straw boaters. They received lessons in etiquette from the school dame. Soon they were taking turns to say grace in Latin before meals in the refectory. The use of native languages was forbidden.

What went for the pupils went also for the masters: they all had to demonstrate a basic knowledge of Latin, irrespective of the subject they were employed to teach. Inevitably this meant hiring everyone from abroad. Indeed, Banda preferred that Malaŵians be employed only as ancillary staff.

The construction of the school was supposedly a gift from the president's own pocket, but the annual running costs consumed almost a third of the national education budget. Regular government schools received on average seventeen US dollars per pupil per year. To educate a child at the academy cost the country 14,000 dollars a year. During an exchange trip, the Head Master of Eton College remarked that Kamuzu Academy was becoming known as 'the Eton of Africa'. But to his mind, he added, Eton should be referred to as 'the Kamuzu Academy of England'.

However, even as the pupils busied themselves with Latin declensions and the Greek definite article, the regime was teetering. Banda had grown very old indeed, and his rule had ossified. The foundation of the academy was a final flourish, followed by a decade of decline. Without much resistance, Banda was toppled in 1994. His one-party state was dismantled and elections were held. He died three years later during the kleptocratic rule of his successor, Bakili Muluzi.

When I arrived in 2009, Malaŵi had just re-elected Bingu wa Mutharika, its second president since Banda. There had been questions about the conduct of the election. The bigger picture was that Bingu presided over the tenth poorest country in the world, a mountain of debt and a budget balanced only by foreign aid; but there had not yet been the calamitous misrule which I would soon witness.

Funding for Kamuzu Academy had stopped abruptly when Banda fell from power. The scholarships were terminated and most of the expatriates departed. To survive, the school had become private. The teachers were now mostly Malaŵians, its pupils the children of 'Big Men' from the capital who could afford the fees.

Amid a wave of nostalgia for the *ancien régime*, Bingu decided to honour Banda's memory by re-establishing a small number of government scholarships. Though the scholars were greatly outnumbered by the private students, the dying embers of Banda's vision flickered briefly to life once more.

III

ARRIVAL

The plane arrived late into Lilongwe, and the sun was already low in the sky. I was picked up by Dr Highbrow, a fellow classicist, now entering his twelfth year at the academy. He hurried me along to minimise time spent travelling in darkness.

Our journey from the capital took us through the central plains, flat and featureless, mile after mile. I remember my surprise that the road signs were identical – in colour, design, typography – to those in England, only they pointed to exotic, unfamiliar places: Kasungu, Mzimba, Nkhotakhota ... It was an odd intrusion of the familiar on the prevailing strangeness.

We were periodically stopped at police checkpoints, our papers inspected by smartly dressed officers in khaki, with peaked caps and swagger sticks. As we waited before the first barrier, two young boys – maybe ten years old – leapt towards us proffering half-a-dozen mice skewered on a stick – a common roadside snack for passing motorists. The animals had been flame-roasted whole, the fur singed off, the tiny bodies charred black and contorted by the heat. When I declined, the boys turned to begging, first for almost worthless coins and then for the empty plastic water bottle in my lap.

We were on the M1, the country's principal motorway,

but it was narrow and pot-holed, disintegrating into dirt track at the edges. Larger vehicles sometimes had to slip off the road altogether to pass each other. Cyclists attempted to cleave unsteadily to the outermost inch of jagged tarmac, the wisest allowing themselves to be driven onto the dirt siding as speeding vehicles skimmed past. Many balanced unwieldy burdens on their panniers: a goat, trussed and bleating; a bale of tobacco; a mother and child. Beside them traipsed an endless line of workers returning from the fields with hoes and machetes. In tiny mud dwellings all around, women kindled innumerable cooking fires that made the failing light hazy with wood smoke.

In between dodging other road users, Dr Highbrow began my initiation into the world of Kamuzu Academy. He spoke with the precision and grandiloquence of a species of don that had almost died out at Oxford.

'It is a fallen institution. The results are execrable. But you will no doubt hear a different account at next week's staff meeting: "Best GCSE results in almost twenty years . . . Ten per cent better than the UK national average . . . More pass grades than ever!" Such speciousness: like listening to figures of tractor production being read out at a meeting of the Supreme Soviet. If the Head Master says it's raining, look out the window, as they say.

'The bright pupils learn stuff; the dim ones do not. There are a few worthy duffers who might be dragged up from an F to a D. But you'll probably find there are better ways to expend your time and energy in Malaŵi. What is worthwhile lies *outside* the academy . . .'

As we drove, the sun set impressively, just as in a tourist brochure, a huge softly glowing circle of deep pink intersected by a sharply defined wisp of horizontal cloud. Darkness then fell abruptly, without the lingering twilight I knew from Europe, and all other traffic melted away. There were no road lights, and, as I tried to trace the outlines of the tarmac, all I could perceive was the cone of our headlights illuminating a void.

But suddenly Dr Highbrow slammed on the brakes, and we screeched to a halt. A few yards further on, a man lay prostrate in the middle of the road. He looked up and, with a flash of a smile, leapt to his feet and trotted away into the darkness. It was winter, and the evening was cold. He had been trying to warm himself on the heat absorbed by the tarmac during the day.

A couple of hours later an elaborately ornamented roundabout appeared out of nowhere, and next we were passing through huge steel gates that bore a crest with the Latin motto *HONOR DEO ET PATRIÆ*. Inside, we were on better tarmac and amid denser vegetation than any we had encountered on our journey. Beside the road were the first street lamps I had seen since leaving the airport access road a hundred miles before. But none was lit – we had arrived at Kamuzu Academy during a power cut.

I ate dinner with Dr Highbrow that night. His villa was well hidden among tall pine trees and dense thickets of bougainvillea. His cook, who had prepared *coq au vin* when the power was on, now reheated it on a clay brazier fired with charcoal. We looked in on his activities and noticed a large dead swamp rat in the kitchen sink. With an awkward smile, the cook summoned a woman from the servant's quarters. She came to the door and received the rodent with a silent curtsy.

The *coq au vin* was tough but flavoursome ('village chicken – to be treated like a game bird') and paired with South African wine ('Allesverloren – all is lost – the name is suited to exile here').

Conversation dwelt on Oxford, where Dr Highbrow had stayed on to complete a doctorate in Wittgensteinian language theory before coming to Malaŵi. He was familiar with several of the dons, and I supplied a little welcome gossip on a few mutual acquaintances.

'Civilisation does still exist there,' Dr Highbrow conceded, 'but only if you know where to find it. A friend of mine who still hangs around in hope of a position calls it "the Cancer Ward". You will find Malaŵi humane after the barbarism of Oxford. What we have here – for now – is a "safe house".'

After dinner, we sat beside the open fire in an imposing living room illuminated by candles wedged into dozens of old wine bottles. Two walls were lined floor to ceiling with books, and a desk was piled high with papers. On the coffee table I noted Plato's *Phaedo*, Frazer's *Golden Bough* and numerous obscure works of local ethnography.

Over whisky, Dr Highbrow spoke as fluently about local custom and contemporary African literature as about epistemology and the Presocratics. It was like being back in an Oxford tutorial room – except that here the walls were hung with a series of monstrous red and black masks that commingled the animal and the human to demonic effect. The flickering light played on their twisted features to suggest still greater malevolence.

'*Gule wamkulu* – the Great Dance,' said Dr Highbrow, noting my distraction. 'It is the supreme cultural achievement of the Chewa people. The masks represent an innumerable pantheon of characters, each with its own moral lesson communicated by a masked dancer. In this way, the wisdom of the ancestors is transmitted down the ages.

'But "representation" does not quite cover it. The dancers are members of a secret society, the Nyau. When they don the masks, they cease to be truly themselves: they *become* the spirits of the ancestors, manifesting themselves as the characters of *gule*. As Mr Sangala explains it when asked directly: "They are dead men who come out of the graves to dance for us."'

'Mr Sangala?'

'Felix Sangala. A man of many parts. And a senior figure in the Nyau. You will no doubt meet him, in due course.'

'And he believes that?'

'The existence of an afterlife is here considered self-evident, the supernatural everywhere inextricable from the real. Only a few weeks ago, a witch aeroplane crashed outside the academy fence.'

'A witch aeroplane?'

'That's right. A couple of passengers broke limbs, but nobody died. Just over the border in Zambia last year, two people were killed in a similar event.'

Dr Highbrow gestured to a broad shallow vessel of woven grass suspended above the fireplace.

'That's a *lichero* – a winnowing basket. It's an object with sinister connotations, and I shouldn't really keep it. But I acquired it early on, and there is now no way of disposing of it that might not arouse even more suspicion. It serves as the cockpit for a witch aeroplane. The witch pilot sits in the basket and steers the craft with a large wooden maize pestle. Some say you need human blood for fuel, but that seems to depend on the wickedness of the witch. Passengers then pay to be transported to otherwise unattainable places: through keyholes, under closed doors, into other people's bedrooms, even abroad.

'The group that crashed recently were musicians from a local band. A passing tourist heard their music and said he would arrange for them to perform in the UK. When he failed to keep his promise, they were understandably disappointed. And so they contracted a witch to convey them to London. Unfortunately they crashed just outside the fence here. I suppose in a delusional state they self-inflict or submit to injury.'

The lights flicked suddenly back on and a cassette player whirred to life with a recording of Bach's *Well-Tempered Clavier*. The power had returned. I felt as if I had understood nothing, my head reeling from fatigue, whisky and the intense weirdness of everything around me. But the irruption of electricity and that warm, humane sound dispelled the unsettling atmosphere. I stepped out onto the veranda and gazed into the immense darkness. There was no moon, and the Milky Way looked like a cache of tiny diamonds scattered onto black velvet. A hyena whooped in the undergrowth, and from far away drifted the faint thud of electronic music.

IV

THE GREAT TRADITION

When Banda died in 1997, I was still at school. The event stirred my head of Classics, Dr Pelion, to recollect the story of the crazed dictator and his academy in the bush. The idea appealed to me, but I did not think of it again for several years.

Within living memory, Classics had been central to my school's ethos. Our Classics library had a venerable old building all of its own, and the Great Hall was emblazoned with the names of classicists dispatched to Oxbridge down the centuries. But when I sat A levels, only two of us took Latin and Greek, instructed in these subjects by four teachers.

Yet it remained an enthusiastic department. Dr Pelion had degrees from both Oxford and Cambridge, and had published a book on Euripides. He elucidated the value of the subject in a way that stuck with me: the modern world was complex and chimerical, ceaselessly changing before our gaze. Greco-Roman culture, on the other hand, was static and remote enough in time to be studied dispassionately. The data was finite and the texts were few, many having been lost in the Dark Ages. The physical remains, like pots and stones and coins, were mostly discovered, catalogued, explained. And of course the languages were dead – that was the whole point. Use could no longer distort them;

the processes of change and decay had been arrested. They possessed the same instructive fixity as the embalmed cadavers I would later study in medical school.

The classical world was a complete microcosm, the richest we possessed. But it was also just small enough that it could be apprehended in totality. Beside the shifting sands of contemporary culture, the Greco-Roman world was a firm and lofty place to stand and survey both past and present. We are all walking blindly into the future, it has been observed. The only difference between us is how far our vision penetrates backwards into the past.

That was Dr Pelion's analysis. But he was no wet-eyed miniature don stepped out of *Goodbye, Mr Chips* or *The Browning Version*. He had taken his doctorate at King's College, Cambridge in a welter of leftist radicalism. He was impassioned in speech, shabby in dress, accompanied by a little white dog and occasionally a faint aroma of marijuana. He was also, it demands to be said, a deeply kind man.

In our final year, he taught us Euripides' last play, *The Bacchae* – the tragedy of King Pentheus, whose repression of primal urges results in his own violent destruction. It was revelatory of a dark savagery concealed beneath the stereotype of Greek culture as lucid, ordered and rational.

Dr Pelion was also responsible for our initiation into the postmodernist approach to the humanities. We learnt that the scholar's real task was 'deconstruction': the stripping away of unconscious bias (our own and the authors') so that the real significance of a text could at last be glimpsed. This seemed exciting at the time, and we went to university brimming with the arcane terminology and precepts of Michel Foucault, Jacques Derrida and Edward Said. It was only later that I would sense a pernicious impulse at work in this.

Classics at Oxford was still known then by its historical title: *Literae Humaniores* or 'more human(e) letters'. The name was meant to draw a distinction with theology and imply that classical literature is so elevated as to fall only just short of the divine. But in my first term I saw an Old Etonian classicist lick cocaine off another's face with the advice: 'You're an animal – act like one.'

Studying Classics produces conflicting feelings. Until recently, the subject had been central to education in the humanities. It was thought to train the mind, furnish wisdom, teach justice and inculcate virtue. But nobody speaks of wisdom and virtue in Oxford today – it would feel unforgivably gauche. As a classicist, you are supposed to hold the keys to 'the best that has been thought and said'. At the same time, however, you are studying something that is repudiated, often contemptuously, by the modern world. In choosing Classics, you arouse the suspicion that you must be mired in the past or otherwise unfit for real life. 'What can you possibly do with that degree?' is repeatedly asked. Defending the subject grows wearisome, and it is easier to retreat into nostalgia or assume a pose of contempt.

A nineteenth-century Oxford don called Gaisford made one of the most infamous claims about Latin and Greek: 'The study of ancient tongues not only refines the intellect and elevates above the common herd but also leads not infrequently to positions of considerable emolument.' This fatuity probably marked the apogee of Classics, with Gaisford epitomising a mentality which would embitter the world against the subject. Immense complacency was followed by protracted decline. Nevertheless, the quotation sticks and might have been better known to many of my contemporaries than any line of Vergil or Homer.

Classics at Oxford felt tired. Students arrived having read a fraction of the texts their predecessors would have done a generation before. Every year, the faculty adapted to decline by cutting down the reading requirements – quite dramatically during the four years I was there. More recently it has even been mooted that Homer and Vergil might be removed from the curriculum altogether.

Ability to write in Latin or Greek had begun to vanish from the university, and the learning of facts, as opposed to opinions, was considered *infra dig* among arts students in general. The best of the dons possessed humane and brilliant minds, but too often they gave the impression of having retreated into small, defensible corners. The only outspoken academics seemed concerned with disclaiming elitism, decolonising the curriculum and celebrating inclusivity through 'outreach' programmes.

Classical scholarship was once highly technical: textual criticism, historical linguistics, mechanisms of oral transmission – these had been the bread and butter of the discipline. But without linguistic proficiency or real faith in the value of the task, such arid challenges are difficult to sustain.

Only the postmodernist school could claim relevance and vitality. Classical texts had to be deconstructed before they could be understood properly as the propaganda of those who wield power. Greece and Rome, it was implied, were the progenitors of the European patriarchy that still exists at every level of our culture. With a postmodernist lens, it is possible to trace the thread of exploitation, racism and misogyny down the millennia from the Bronze Age in Greece to the present day. The classicist's main duty is to sift the inheritance for evidence of guilt.

This approach makes life easy from the undergraduate point of view, as the rubric can be learnt in five minutes and then applied to everything. The conclusions have been reached already: the authors and their white male confrères were the oppressors; women, slaves and foreigners the oppressed. Any mention of an oppressed group could be read as evidence of this, as could any failure to mention them. There is probably not a classicist in the country who hasn't written about about Vergil's portrayal of women in a spirit of lip service to feminist ideology, or about Herodotus's colonialising purpose in studying the Persians. A few students bring fresh zeal to this work, especially if they hope to pursue careers in academia. But for most it is a convenient way to get through the chore of essays and tutorials. If you played the game and reproduced the right arguments, it was difficult not to pass your exams.

Things might have changed, but, in the mid 2000s, the real energies of Oxford humanities students were expended on dissipation. Barely a day went by without moderate to heavy drinking, which dulled faculties and emboldened opinions, as we staggered about boorishly in silk scarves and evening tails. Drinking like this necessitated long periods of daytime convalescence, perhaps in a college garden with a volume of Tibullus on which to rest your head. Few of the arts students with whom I caroused did much work. The scientists might have suspected this, but our self-confidence was imperturbable and went unchallenged.

The value of the subject was difficult to uphold under these circumstances and, in the final year, cynicism triumphed. Representatives of the big City law firms and finance houses infiltrated our well-heeled binges, laying on lavish networking events which at first we disdained but slowly began to frequent out of interest in the free drinks.

'Have you ever thought about a career in financial consultancy?'

'I'm sorry – this is *cava*,' spluttered the undergraduate in an explosive spray. 'We need to get out of here and find a proper drink.'

It was disconcerting to note that the votaries at these events were undismayed by our petulance. They persisted with Mephistophelian calm until theirs was an accepted presence among the balls, cocktail parties and dining clubs. For four years we had pranced without a care in the world, as if the party would never end. But the more alert began to sense that the ship was foundering – and the corporate world seemed to offer a life-raft.

'You'd be surprised. Oxbridge Classics grads are well regarded in the City. They have a lot of transferable skills . . .'

I recoiled and looked for work abroad – which is how I found myself in Malaŵi.

V

RARE BIRDS

In fierce sunlight Kamuzu Academy shimmers like a mirage against the brilliant blue sky. A mass of bold red brickwork, its architecture nods to the classical vernacular but is otherwise defiantly modern, elegant and oddly congruent with its surroundings of lush tropical greenery. Before the entrance, an ornamental lake is swathed with irises and lilies that gleam purple and gold. The columns of a portico plunge into mirror-like water between banks of papyrus roosted by the sacred ibis.

The gardens and forest have now reached full maturity, an oasis in contrast with the bare central plains outside. With his taste for anomaly, Banda had the grounds planted with exotic trees imported from abroad. This had the unexpected consequence that rare birds are today attracted to the academy in the course of their migration routes. On occasion, the place is sought out by intrepid ornithologists.

The school seemed imposing, but, as I got closer, I noticed missing window panes and long meandering cracks in the masonry. The school bells were silent, and the clocktower told the wrong time. In the Classics department, yellowing posters of the Forum and Acropolis flapped in the breeze that blew through broken louvers. Tattered journals, souvenir guides and OHP slides of archaeological sites teetered in heaps on buckling shelves. Mountains of Greek and Latin texts contained bookplates inscribed with pupils' names, testifying to generations of use brought abruptly to an end.

At the time of my arrival, Classics endured but in a greatly diminished form. All pupils still had to study one ancient language to fifth-form level, with the odd consequence that the school entered more Greek GCSE candidates than anywhere else in the world. But this policy was regarded by most as an unfathomable atavistic reflex. Only a few engaged seriously with the subjects, and the response of many was complete bafflement.

Teaching was complicated by a dichotomy observable between the small cohort of government scholars and the majority fee-paying students. Most of the former came from conditions of poverty, and had performed exceptionally in their entrance exams. The latter were from wealthy families, their fathers belonging to the class identified elsewhere in Africa as *wabenzi*, after their predilection for German limousines.

In the first few years, the scholars worked furiously while the rich pupils too often did very little. Ekari came from a village in the south, where his family were subsistence farmers. You could ask him for the first-person plural pluperfect active subjunctive of the Latin verb 'to love', and he would snap back the answer immediately: *amavissemus*. Beside him slouched Hellington, the son of a member of parliament. At age thirteen, he could barely write his own name. It should be observed, however, that the two sat together in perfect amity. On the rare occasions that Hellington was stirred to make an effort, he would prevail upon his friend to produce a piece of homework for him, and Ekari would cheerfully comply.

There was no streaming, so at first, half the class got full marks while the rest struggled to answer a single question.

Such absurd conditions tempted a cynical response. But, for all he might say to his colleagues, Dr Highbrow was a dedicated and humane schoolmaster. He set an example of patience, humour and kindliness, and the pupils adored him.

'Now, children, we are at Book Four, line 365 of Vergil's *Aeneid*. Dido is angry – Right, come in, both of you, you're late. And Hellington, why are you looking like a dustbin? Dress yourself, boy, or you can go to Mr Machila's office, and he will put your *machende* in the Magimix.

'Where was I? Dido is angry with Aeneas. She denies that Venus is his mother and that Dardanus is the founder of his race. Thank you, Ekari, that is indeed why we call the Trojans *Dardanidae*. Yes, that's correct, a patronymic – well spotted.

'Now, we need a subject, something in the nominative. Well done, Prudence: *tigres*. Now what are *tigres*? Hellington, wake up, boy! You can pay homage to catatonia during break. *Tigres* sounds like . . . Sounds like . . . ? No? Ah, thank you for putting us out of our misery, Mtendere: tigers.

'And now the tigers need a verb. It's got to be plural . . . Well done, Godwin: *admorunt*. Err, yes, thank you, Ekari, that is indeed a poetic contraction . . . Yes, perfect active indicative, that's right.

'So: "tigers moved something towards you". (Don't be frightened, Nelly. "You" is Aeneas.) And what is that something? What did they move? We need an object, Matalina: find the accusative! Very good: *ubera*. And what are *ubera*? I can give you a clue: something to do with milk. Where do mothers store their milk?

'No! Not in the fridge, Salome dear! That's what the mothers of the *azungu* do, and we all know how *their* children grow up.

'*Ubera*? Can nobody translate *ubera*?!'

'BREASTS, boys and girls! Breasts, udders, nipples, knockers, teats, titties, you name it. So: "tigers moved their udders towards you". She is calling Aeneas a beast, claiming he must have been suckled by tigers . . . OK, thank you, Ekari, "tigresses" might be better English . . .'

The ludicrous disparity did not matter so much in the early years. The problem was that, as they entered their teens, the rich pupils set the tone and the scholars began to emulate their attitude and behaviour. Results converged at the bottom and typically reached a nadir as everyone approached A level.

Motivation was easily undermined because prospects on leaving school were so poor. After the chimerical world of the academy, they faced the reality of life in one of the world's weakest economies. Further study was possible only for the few. Jobs were scarce and seemed too often the gift of those with power, rather than won by merit. I remember some scholars who might have made it to Oxbridge had they been living in the UK. At the end of the sixth form they returned to their parents' smallholdings to resume the occupation descriptively termed 'just staying'.

The possibility of material success seemed fantastically remote. Where it was occasionally observed, it seemed to have been won by a process of lottery. It is, after all, in Malaŵi that Madonna sporadically scatters largesse and has adopted four children. Besides this, you might be noticed by a passing football talent scout, marry a foreign tourist or hit the jackpot through the caprice of political election. The profits of any of these were spectacular compared with what might be earned by actual work.

Such a perverse situation threw into question the whole purpose of education. But it also liberated teaching from the utilitarian concerns which can stifle learning back in the UK. There was no hoop-jumping, point-scoring, CV-polishing or other cynical behaviour. Nor did ambitious parents agitate about exam tactics or the canniest way to submit a UCAS form. For those who wished to engage, study was primarily its own reward.

Expatriate teachers came and went frequently, but there was a small core of Oxbridge Classics graduates who were committed to a long exile. Their frame of mind was resolutely academic – a reproach to me after my own university experience. They pursued interests seeded during their degrees but redirected towards the local culture and invigorated by it. They read Greek and Latin seriously but also learnt Malaŵi's languages and brought to them the philologist's attentiveness. They observed customs, compiled dictionaries, catalogued art, transcribed oral traditions, filmed dance and recorded music. The country had won their hearts, and they would speak informedly and with a cultivated partiality about its history and prehistory, flora and fauna, peoples and gods.

Their interests led them outside the academy compound and into a world wildly different from their own. In my first term I observed colleagues set aside their Greek lexicons to supervise the harvest at experimental farms, count heads of elephant and antelope in the nearby game reserve, source steel girders for a bridge in the national park and convey quantities of cement down unspeakable roads to construct schools in distant villages. They bothered local artists and transacted unfathomable business with village headmen. You might have suspected they were simply bored, but the contrary was the case. The peculiarity of the situation and their unlimited freedom fanned enthusiasms that had only smouldered back at home.

Their conversation was witty and inventive but could slide into cattishness and snobbery as they lambasted colleagues and, especially, each other. One of Dr Highbrow's fussier fellow classicists was ridiculed for his 'galloping hypochondria', and his obsession with lists, inventories, mark readjustment, and the height of pupils' desks. 'The List Fairy's at it again: snuffing about those f---ing desks like a prize poodle with a pine cone up its arse!'

Another teacher who dozed through an exam invigilation was 'sat on his fat arse doing the square root of bugger all – about as much use as a dildo in an abattoir!'

Unhelpful colleagues became evidence of the academy's 'equal opportunity employment policy: not to discriminate on the grounds of inability or disinclination to do their job'.

'It'll be affirmative action next: that means seeking out complete retards.'

Careerists among the teaching staff were at risk of contracting 'Hepatitis A of the brain – from all that arse-licking of the board of governors'.

'Middle management' in general was 'evidence of metastasis of the primary lesion'.

Pupils were spared unkindness, but the dimmer ones were regarded pityingly: 'He's a nice little boy but he's got a hardware problem. It's no use blaming sydelxia – the processing capacity simply isn't there.'

The shortcomings of the academy brought out an acid cynicism, but when pupils emerged who wanted to engage, Dr Highbrow's response was serious and dedicated. For these, teaching was conducted after school in small groups sometimes drawn from different years, and there was an atmosphere of cabbalistic intrigue about it.

The boarding houses were ungovernable. On approach, you were assailed by a continuous roar of disorder and a stifling odour of *chamba* smoke and uncleanliness. An evening inspection was conducted as briefly as possible – like a peace-keeping force that knows its own impotence in a hostile land. Then responsibility for a semblance of good order was delegated to prefects and a guard in army fatigues who kept a muzzled attack-dog precariously tethered to his chair leg. He kept watch outside sturdy locked gates for the rest of the night.

Behind these, at the appointed time, a small party of classicists would sidle up, wielding Homeric dictionaries or Latin primers. The senior house master might convey crapulous approval by telephone from the club bar and the pupils would be let through. We teachers gathered with them in deserted classrooms and worked by candlelight if the sun had set and there was a power cut. The evening air hung heavy with the scent of frangipani as we discussed texts, practised Latin prose composition, or declaimed lines of Homer, sending up rolling hexameters into the immense silent darkness.

It was not, in fact, completely useless. Greek and Latin are difficult, and I suspect many pupils got more mental exercise from these than they did from a lot of other subjects. The languages are highly inflected, the grammar and syntax strict and complex, the idiom remote. You need to think logically and systematically, but also imaginatively. And you have to develop deep powers of memory. It was gratifying to observe how, the more pupils learnt, the faster they could learn more. Their knowledge snowballed, their understanding deepened, and their articulation in English improved noticeably. Latin and Greek were certainly no less useful for most than learning about quadratic equations, ox-bow lakes or other staples of 'more practical' subjects.

But there was more to it than this. In Europe now, we cannot approach ancient texts without the skepticism and neuroses of modernity. Too much has happened, and we look back on antiquity through the miasma of history, our judgement clouded by centuries of disputatious commentary.

But these pupils seemed able to engage with the texts more directly and ingenuously. There was no single response that was revelatory, just a general impression that they could take what they read at face value in a way that I could not.

When I also took a sixth-form class for English literature, the contrast was instructive. T.S. Eliot's *The Waste Land* was the set text that year, and I agreed to help a Malaŵian colleague. He was a nice man who conscientiously studied the Bible, but I sensed that he had never read a book for pleasure. He spent a lot of time hawking samosas in the boys' hostels.

Only two pupils were taking the paper, both worthy. I was eager to see how they would respond, but it was not a great success. *The Waste Land* is a work of 1920s Modernism, and its gloomy enigmatic meditation on twenty centuries of history, books and broken images seemed irrelevant. Only the biblical allusions did they identify instantly – often before I had picked up on them myself.

To a lesser degree, it was the same with Auden, Tennyson, Byron, Donne. I had always cherished the faith that these were universal and could speak to any place or time. But I became conscious of the essential European-ness of so much English literature – even Shakespeare. *Macbeth* and *King Lear* have crossed enormous gulfs. But the moody individualism of *Hamlet* jarred in Malaŵi. And the equivocal moral assizes of *Measure for Measure* were just very obscure.

In contrast, there was a robust directness to classical literature. And in Malaŵi you might every day encounter the figures that populated the worlds of its authors. The pastoral poetry of Hesiod and Vergil had meant nothing to me at university. But for many of these pupils, the livelihoods of goatherds and crofters were a familiar reality.

Classicists in Europe might spend a lifetime straining to

understand the warrior code of Homer. In Malaŵi, though mostly vanished, an analogous culture lingered on in the martial rituals of the Ngoni, who still danced with spears and shields that Achilles would have known how to use.

As for the sanguinary horrors of Greek tragedy, I came to realise how faintly they echoed in my own genteel world. When I was at school, I could only test out precocious opinions about the Oedipus Complex. But in these classes, I could illustrate the stories of Aeschylus, Sophocles and Euripides with clippings from the daily newspapers: 'Malaŵi's Infanticide Shame', 'Impalement in Karonga', 'Elephant Gores Six in Liwonde', 'Vampire Menace Strikes Again' . . .

In general, the supernatural and the polytheistic needed no post-Enlightenment gloss. When the witch Circe turned Odysseus's men into swine, I made a weak joke about the fate that might befall those who failed their vocab tests. My listeners fell into a reproachful silence. Eventually, one girl spoke up solemnly from the back: 'Sir. You mustn't say things like that.'

It was a chastening moment. But it was from these classes that I had my first intimation that the classical world and the Malaŵian village might be closer to each other in spirit than either was to our own modern way of life. And that this was not because of any shortcoming in the local culture. It was because we in the West had become alienated from something elemental and important.

VI

THE VILLAGE

The Village – not a particular village or even a single place, but rather the world inhabited by the overwhelming majority of Malaŵi's population. Of course they live *in* villages, as others do – but there is more to this than the places and physical structures. It is a mode of being and belonging whose every activity is recognisable and meaningful to those who know it.

There was a small hill where villagers sometimes went to pray, and, at its foot, stood a tiny chapel of mud-brick and thatch. The interior was orderly, the atmosphere serene. It had no altar, but a rough wooden cross hung on the wall before six neat mounds of earth smoothed by hand into pews.

Scrambling up the hill, I could peer down into three or four tidy villages. The huts were also mud and grass but each had a little *khonde*, or porch, on which old men took their ease together. In the shade of mango trees, young women pounded maize and gossiped. Dogs slept in compounds marked out by tightly woven reed fences. A brook burbled in a nearby gulley where a father was teaching boys to fish. Downstream, some girls were teasing each other as they lay freshly washed clothes on a broad flat stone to dry. Above them, on the hill, a shepherd sat singing on a log as his flock grazed around him. In the surrounding fields, the harvest was in and farmers leant on their hoes, consorting over trails of late pumpkins ripening between rows of withered cornstalks. Beside me, a pair of rock dassies emerged from their holes to sniff among the wild flowers.

It was an idyll such as Theocritus might have known, but its life was also harsh and precarious. Malaŵi is poor and densely populated. Its 20 million people suffer progressively with land shortage as their population grows and they try to subsist on smallholdings and a single annual maize crop.

Farmers plant with the first rains and reap six to eight months later. Then everyone waits patiently to see if the harvest will be sufficient unto the next. So much hangs on the government's annual fertiliser handout. There is little irrigation to support a second growing season, minimal crop diversification and often no access to any cash economy.

Fields are tilled entirely by hand, and almost everything, from bricks to water, is carried on the head over immense distances. Very few villagers have access to bicycles; fewer still to a cart improvised from wood and broken auto-parts, usually pulled by an emaciated ox. The issue of transport – for any purpose whatever – is a perpetual, even existential problem. Public minibuses are few, irregular, dangerous and expensive. Ownership of a private vehicle is rare and the distinguishing mark of a man who has risen from the village and acquired 'status'. For everyone else, life is lived almost entirely within walking distance of the place they were born.

Most years, life drifts by uneventfully. Boys hang about in idle throngs, occasionally seeking out piece-work. The girls have children – as many as half before they are eighteen. Catastrophe is part of the routine. Every few years some blight, dearth, drought or famine sweeps the land, taking with it the old, the young, the infirm and the unlucky. And even in years of plenty, every family is individually vulnerable to all the natural shocks that flesh is heir to.

Still, there was resilience and vitality in the face of hardship, and somehow even good cheer. I could never prove this or quantify it, but I felt it every day in a myriad of warm and generous gestures. It was present in villagers' indefatigable courtesy, in the laughter that met any inconvenience and in the smiles that defied privation. It was a nebulous thing to describe, yet obvious and striking when observed. Indeed, it was often the first thing visitors remarked upon.

'What is worthwhile here lies *outside* the academy' had been Dr Highbrow's remark on my arrival. I sensed that he was right, but it felt difficult to engage deeply with the world of the village. I could walk into it easily enough and receive a delightful welcome, but the encounter remained superficial.

My first opportunity for more meaningful contact came through Flemings Chaseka, a quiet and dignified Chewa man nearing sixty whom I employed as a 'houseboy/cookboy' – these terms still being endemic in Malaŵi and applied even to men in advanced old age. He had worked for the *azungu* – foreigners, white people – for almost two decades, more often than not for Classics teachers from whom he had acquired a stack of eloquent references.

Servants make us uneasy, and my English guests sometimes deplored the arrangement. But through Flemings, I gained an entry into lives that would otherwise have remained remote. I was familiar with cleaners in London who might come once or twice a week and were expected to interact as little as possible. The premium virtue was invisibility – to be trustworthy enough to work while the employer was out. The arrangement in Malaŵi could not have been more different: Flemings was there all the time. At first, this irritated me, and I never ceased to feel slightly self-conscious if I were idle in the same room while he worked. But he brought warmth to a house that would otherwise have been lonely. My spirits came to soar at the exuberance with which he said 'Good morning!' or greeted me after work: 'Good evening, *bwana*! Tonight you will please be eating . . .' – Flemings would here sustain a dramatic pause for as long as he dared – ' . . . sausages!'

There were of course odd occasions of discord, but, for the most part, his good spirits were irrepressible. I felt ashamed at how much gloom I could bring to my work when I encountered him singing merrily at his sweeping. He possessed the Elixir of George Herbert's poem that could 'make drudgery divine'.

His salary was nugatory, the relationship was all. It was the basis for appeal in the myriad crises that beset his family: a lift to the hospital when his daughter was convulsing with eclampsia, the ensuing medical bills, the cost of a new roof when his mother's house was wrecked by heavy rain, his father's funeral expenses. These and a thousand lesser requests could chafe. But the dependency involved me in his whole life, and I had a stake in his prosperity as well as in his hardship. I knew of his son's success in getting a job in the town, of his mother's unexpected recovery from tuberculosis, of his eldest daughter's marriage. And there was inter-dependency too, as when I had malaria and Flemings kept watch over me in my delirium.

He had a large family and provided for them from his wages and a tiny patch of land. It was a fragile existence, and he had been out of work for some time when I employed him. He wore his best clothes to 'interview', and they were clean but tattered. So I could only marvel when a widowed cousin of his died and he unhesitatingly adopted her two young children, the boy less than a year old. He had of course found relative prosperity in working for me. But the two extra mouths to feed were a considerable burden, and he would have no cash income whenever I left Malaŵi.

'But can you afford to look after them, Flemings?' I asked doubtfully.

'These children – they have no one now!' he answered, quite cheerfully.

The *non sequitur* suggested an instinctual and unquestioning generosity. It was my first observation of an attitude towards children that regarded them as an unqualifiedly good thing, to be rejoiced in whatever the circumstances, like an abundant harvest.

Flemings was a figure of some standing in the village. There was prestige associated with being a household servant, but he was also renowned as a man of experience. Stories circulated of his snatching the honey of forest bees with his bare hands, and he had once bludgeoned to death a ferocious wild pig with a golf club. When the dog shooter, Chief Hunter Phiri, visited the academy to destroy vermin, I asked Flemings if he knew him.

'Yes. I know Chief Hunter Phiri. And Chief Hunter Phiri knows me.' This was confirmed when the legendary hunter appeared on my *khonde* with his old army beret and Lee-Enfield .303 to greet his friend. But Flemings took care to keep my dog tethered in the yard for the duration of his stay – an alarming week during which deafening reports would sound at random immediately outside my classroom window and festering canine corpses gathered under the bushes, the wounded strays having crawled there to bleed to death.

When we had occasion to travel north, we visited Flemings' parents. I was assured they lived close to the main road, but it turned out to be a long diversion down narrow tracks, overgrown and choked by sand. I resented the inconvenience and grumbled, but my mood softened when at length we reached their residence. Cassava was densely planted all around, and one wall of the house was adorned with a flowering creeper. Yet the building itself seemed on the point of tumbling down. Everywhere cracks were spreading and the lower half of each wall was discoloured and friable with rot. The mud had once been whitewashed, but only traces of this now remained. The roof was sagging, the door frame ready to buckle. The couple who emerged were haggard, stooped and thin, the husband leaning on his wife's shoulder and coughing unobtrusively. Still they welcomed us with bright, smiling eyes and infinite grace.

'Hello, how are you?' they each asked in turn.

'I am fine, thank you. What about you?'

'I am also fine, thank you.'

'Thank you.'

So goes the universal formulaic greeting in Malaŵi. The words are clunking and seem at first inconsequential. But they may be the only English known to many, and their use is totally ubiquitous. Not to participate in the exchange is considered very rude, and this principle is upheld to the point of stoic absurdity. I would later meet desperately sick patients in hospital who would reassure me that they were 'fine, thank you' and enquire after my own health before expiring in front of me. Dr Highbrow had even once witnessed a village Passion Play which assumed the same prosaic exchange to have taken place between Christ and Pontius Pilate before the crucifixion. There was something telling in this defiant, laboured striving after courtesy. It suggested an absolute dedication to the principle that 'manners makyth man', and reminded me of T.S. Eliot when he defined tradition as 'All those habitual actions, habits, and customs, from the most significant religious rite to our conventional way of greeting a stranger, which represent the blood kinship of "the same people living in the same place".'

We sat down to eat. The Chasekas had borrowed chairs from neighbours and had arranged them in the shade of an aged guava tree close by the *khonde*. We were joined by other family members, but the frail mother still insisted on laying out the dishes she had prepared while her daughter knelt beside me with a vessel of water to douse my hands before eating. An array of dented lidless pots with broken handles contained tepid thickset maize porridge, gritty cassava pap, woody greens and – a luxury for them – boiled tripe, stinking and turgid in a little greasy scum. The women sat in the dust, waiting as the men ate and foisting more on us whenever possible. It was a memorably disgusting meal, but I buried this feeling in shame before their immense generosity. They gave with joy and ate with gratitude. It could not have been more different to the impatient privilege and discontented security which I knew. I felt it as a reproach to my whole way of being.

VII

YOUR PROTOTYPE

Through Flemings, my acquaintance with the village widened, and I decided to rent a small patch of farmland for myself. It would furnish vegetables for the kitchen, but the greater part would be dedicated to tobacco, Malaŵi's principal cash crop. I thought the sale might offset some of the costs of the farm, but I was mainly interested just to find out how it was grown.

The land was about ten miles from the academy and reached only by a faint, tortuous track on which I never saw another vehicle. It was poor, stony land, far from any village, but it sloped down into a marsh where water could be drawn. It was owned by a minor chief who also worked as a cook in the academy kitchens. He had several tenant farmers living there, and they would grow the tobacco. I took them with the land on a one-year contract, paying them for their labour in cash but also with foot-long bars of soap and razor blades. This seemed an unduly complicated process of remuneration until I realised that, to buy their own, they would have to travel thirty miles to the nearest town – an expensive journey. I could pick up soap and razors whenever I passed through in my car. These were the only products they demanded of the outside world.

Senior among the tenants was Lysard Moyo. His first name had, I think, been invented to satisfy my interest, and neither he nor the landowner could pronounce it consistently. Both were illiterate in any language, but the landowner spoke fair English. Lysard Moyo communicated very little. He lived at the edge of the plot in a dilapidated hut so low you could not stand upright inside it. His only window was sealed with a piece of rotting board. The roof was grass, reinforced here and there with scraps of plastic bag weighed down with stones. He occupied the hut with a family of six, although I believe a nearby trench in the ground covered with a fragment of tarpaulin served as an extra room.

He had rough features, a patchy hispid beard and an unsettlingly vacant expression. For clothing he possessed a single torn orange shirt, always soiled, and a length of coarse fabric which hung from his loins. But it was his strength that seemed to define him. He hunched awkwardly from years of carrying immense burdens but was still tall and possessed perhaps the broadest shoulders I have ever seen. He could wield a hoe or mattock not only forcefully but with an awesome efficiency. I would watch in feeble astonishment as he turned row after row of rock and clay as if it were the lightest compost, or felled in minutes with his blunt axe a tree that would have cost me hours, and probably an injury. There was a surprising niftiness to him too, as when he cradled uprooted tobacco seedlings in his palm before replanting them in the soil he had uplifted. Everything turned green with his touch.

From a small bed of weed-like sprouts, Lysard Moyo brought forth acres of brilliant emerald-green tobacco, so dense and high that his children would play hide-and-seek in it. The whole family then picked the big, supple leaves and hung them to dry in long sheds he had constructed from sticks and branches bound with jute. The tobacco began to glow gold as it dried, whereupon it was pressed into bales and stacked up in every corner of my living room, filling the house with its sapid, grown-up smell.

Mrs Moyo was also formidably built and every day walked miles back and forth from the well with gallons of potable water on her head in the family's treasured plastic jerry can. I seldom observed more than a single word pass between her and her husband, and once I saw him snarl sullenly, causing her to recoil as if in fear of his reach. But she was tender with her children, instructing them so they might contribute to the task of survival, the girls by building fires and drawing water, the boys by carrying rocks and working the soil with digging sticks.

And survive they did. You might judge these people the wretched of the earth and, as I would soon see for myself, their existence was tragically vulnerable. But there was more to it than that. They were wrenching life itself from that inhospitable ground, and Lysard Moyo defied a cruel and fickle universe to feed and multiply his family. They faced terrible odds with great courage. And in their will to impose order on the chaos of nature, there was a lofty humanity.

They were peasants through and through, of the sort that has almost entirely vanished from our midst in Europe. An Irish missionary told me how Malaŵi reminded him of his boyhood in County Kerry when the land was still tilled by hand. But tractors had been introduced there when he was a young man and life soon changed beyond recognition. His elderly mother had made one visit to him in Africa, and he related how moved she had been to feel quite at home among its people.

For my part, I could only turn to books that had hitherto meant nothing to me. Lysard Moyo might have stepped out of any of the pastoral literature of Greece and Rome, from Hesiod's *Works and Days* or from Vergil's *Georgics* or

Eclogues. But it was the poem 'A Peasant', by the twentieth-century Welshman R.S. Thomas, that best described him and his kinship to me.

> [. . .] see him fixed in his chair
> Motionless, except when he leans to gob in the fire
> There is something frightening in the vacancy of his mind.
> His clothes, sour with years of sweat
> And animal contact, shock the refined,
> But affected, sense with their stark naturalness.
> Yet this is your prototype, who, season by season
> Against siege of rain and the wind's attrition,
> Preserves his stock, an impregnable fortress
> Not to be stormed even in death's confusion.
> Remember him, then, for he, too, is a winner of wars,
> Enduring like a tree under the curious stars.

At Oxford, I had studied the Roman poet Vergil and his great epic, *The Aeneid*. Its subject is war in the most literal sense, but the rest of Vergil's poetry is about farming, and it had always perplexed me why he should have fastened upon two such different themes. Now, however, seeing the heroism of such 'winners of wars' as Lysard Moyo, the connection made perfect sense.

VIII

CULTURE WARS

The village adjacent to Kamuzu Academy was called Mtunthama, and it sprawled along the estate's perimeter fence and tarmac access road. It possessed a dozen or more concrete structures, including a post office built under Banda, a prosperous 'boozing parlour' known as Edgar's Beehive Club and Auntie Kay's – an establishment against which I was sternly warned. There was a fuel station that seldom had any fuel, and a clinic that seldom had any drugs. The 'Boyz 2 Men Welding Shop' was not, Dr Highbrow observed, a pederastic supply agency. And I was disinclined to purchase meat from the 'Butchery', where a fly-blown carcass was suspended from a tripod of sticks, twisting slowly in the sun. Beside these enterprises, there were several churches, a mosque and a teeming jumble of mud-brick houses.

A tall steel gate asserted the divide between village and academy, and a worker in army fatigues saluted as you passed between them. But while the gate was forbidding, the fence was highly permeable. It had once been maintained and patrolled by soldiers of the Malawi Defence Force; now it was rusted and frayed, with so many holes that a constant traffic of visitors flowed in and out to conduct covert and inscrutable business. During the day, vendors with unaccountable bundles of wares might be loitering importunately outside your house. Driving back late one night, my headlights startled a party of foragers poking at something in a tree with a big stick. Dr Highbrow was once robbed as he walked home through the estate at dusk.

Yet he in particular upheld the goal of bringing together village and academy. It was not really the gate or the fence that divided them, but rather psychological barriers, which often felt unbreachable.

Over several years, Dr Highbrow had collected extensive footage of local dances, and he tried showing some to his tutorial group. The attention of the poorer pupils was immediately captured, as if by something important but recently forgotten. For a moment, they were as engaged as the village children watching in the background of the film. But then they detected the sneers of the cool kids who sat at the back of the classroom gazing into iPhones. They became self-conscious of their peasant ways and attempted to play down their interest.

In 1971, Landeg White, a contributor to the Malaŵian poetry anthology *Mau*, made a mordant comment on the meeting of local and Western cultures:

> In the village
> A deep debate:
> The chief's daughter has a transistor;
> She is dancing to the Beatles
> Gaily outside her hut.
> But the tape-recorder man
> On his codification project wants
> 'Your own music,' he demands,
> 'Marimba! Bangwe!'
> The chief is bemused
> By this pressure from Europe
> Not to attend to Europe:

Is he 'himself'
With the radio on or off?

The poem captures much of the tension and irony in Dr Highbrow's efforts with his class, but I couldn't help feeling that the cultural dissonance had evolved considerably since White's day.

Each school house had an annual celebratory dinner to which pupils were allowed to wear their own clothes. The fee-paying pupils would arrive bathed in fragrance and immodestly attired, the boys conforming to the 'gangster rap' style – oversized basketball shirts and sagging pants, fake gold chains and fanciful sunglasses, loping gaits copied from MTV; the girls were usually over-painted and under-dressed.

The government scholars presented themselves very differently. They would enter meekly, dressed with care in shabby outfits assembled from their village clothes. The girls were often in a monochrome 'Sunday best' dress obviously sown by amateur hands. A few boys, lacking anything smarter, wore their school uniform. And all of them huddled out of the limelight in which their wealthier peers disported themselves triumphantly.

It was the fee-paying pupils' style of dress, with its associated music, idiolect and culture, to which almost everyone – pupils, teachers, Big Men, even wealthier peasants – seemed to aspire. This aesthetic glittered from satellite TV and the Internet. Its sounds thundered from car stereos and grated from the tinny speakers of cell-phones. Its costume could be bought off the back of a truck bearing cheap imports from Durban or Dar es Salaam. It was a vision of bling, enchanting because it was felt to emanate from black, not white, America. Perhaps it did – but it was also fundamentally Western and commercial, and it eclipsed everything in the village, which lacked status by comparison. The music was supposed to have its roots in Africa. True or not, the local culture seemed to wither on contact with it.

Perhaps classicists are trained to be hypersensitive to the erosion of tradition. Certainly, colleagues from other departments seemed unconcerned by this phenomenon. Many of the Malaŵian staff were preoccupied with small businesses which they had capitalised with their academy salary. This was hardly surprising as their prosperity frequently attracted so many dependants that they had to subsidise their incomes however they could. But what leisure time they had seemed all too often given over to television, football, and – in many cases – drink.

The approach to alcohol was binary: you either drank or you did not. And if you did, you drank stolidly and tirelessly to achieve catatonia. This process might start with Carlsberg and South African brandy but would then decline into Powers Number One Spirit – a product of the Dwangwa ethanol factory, sold in the sort of small plastic sachets used for condiments in UK fast food restaurants. When the money ran really low, drinkers turned to *kachasu* – the maleficent local moonshine. Binges started promptly on payday and lasted until the money ran out – whereupon sobriety was good-naturedly resumed. A pupil once complained meekly to me that one of her teachers had been drunk all week. I asked if this had at least been amusing. Yes, but only at first, she replied. Now it was just boring. I felt rebuked for asking such a frivolous question.

Of course, there was even heavier drinking among most expatriates, but their intake tended to be steadier and so less disruptive. This was probably because they were better able to fund it, being paid double the salary of their Malaŵian counterparts. Most exhibited little curiosity in their surroundings. They occupied themselves with sport, drinking games and bullying locals.

After Banda's fall, expatriates could only be employed if no Malaŵian possessed the formal qualifications for the job. This had the odd result that, apart from Classics, only the more novel subjects were taught by foreigners, as no teacher training existed for these locally.

So apart from the small core of classicists, the British population included a Glaswegian business studies teacher, who was to be found wrecked on gin every night at the club, sometimes sobbing into her glass. She was sacked only after she was caught having *group* sex with her sixth form. Her closest ally taught design and technology: he was regularly so drunk he had to be carried home by security staff, though they gave up on this when he locked them in a garage and had them beg for their lives on bended knee while he wielded a panga knife about their heads.

Engagement between most expatriates and village Malaŵians was usually limited. Some might kick around a football with local players. For others, there were occasional excursions to a nearby orphanage to cuddle babies and pose for photos. A few entered into relationships with Malaŵians, and it could be touching to see the civilising effects of this contact. But the liaisons were usually short-lived.

A PE teacher from the UK confessed she had only rarely sat down to dinner at table before coming to Malaŵi. Now every day she paused before eating as her Malaŵian boyfriend said grace. But, in the end, it was the mores of the UK that prevailed. She had spoken openly about how much she wanted 'a little black baby' and, after only a few months in the country, she got pregnant and left, citing her need to give birth in a British hospital. She never returned, and cut off contact with the dismayed father. He was a decent man, but it was inconceivable that he might find the means to move abroad, or even visit, without her support.

I asked Flemings what he thought about all this, but he was too polite to comment.

IX

GRADUS AD PARNASSUM

It has been contended that the classical education fosters narrow-mindedness, introspection, Eurocentricism. At the academy, however, a small number of long-staying classicists exhibited an obsessive curiosity in the unfamiliar society around them. Dr Highbrow, in particular, sought to combine the best that both village and academy had to offer. He raised funds to construct local schools and lured academy pupils out to teach in them. He led a volunteer programme which got others to decorate a church and build a clinic. He presided over a Duke of Edinburgh scheme that ran expeditions deep into the bush. Above all, he turned to drama, enlisting both the academy and various humbler village institutions into the international Shakespeare Schools Festival. But it was in his productions of Greek theatre that he really hoped to achieve a meeting of worlds.

The Bacchae is Euripides' last play, written at the end of the fifth century BC, while he was in exile from his native Athens in the wilds of Macedonia. It concerns the arrival of Dionysus, originally a foreign deity and the last to join the Greek pantheon. He is the god of wine and madness, dance, theatre, and the mask. He is to be worshipped with revelry in remote places, far outside the city walls. Women, not men, lead the rites that assume the form of orgiastic frenzy.

Social barriers dissolve, the earth yields wine and honey, and all creatures, even the fiercest, consort harmoniously with man. The object of the revelry, as an Oxford don wrote, is to recover the potency of animal being, liberate the instincts, attain a strange new vitality and commune with the god, your fellow worshippers and the whole life of the earth.

King Pentheus resists this innovation, deploring the moral licence sanctioned by Dionysus, whom he rejects, appealing instead to reason and sobriety. But as the whole city, including his mother and sisters, cavort off into the mountains, he is overwhelmed by prurience and sneaks after them to watch. His family catch him spying but fail to recognise him: lost in ecstasy and intoxication, they tear his body limb from limb with their bare hands and devour his raw flesh. The tale has been interpreted as a reminder that dark impulses can never be fully repressed. The Greeks championed lucidity and self-control, but Euripides reminded them that release from these constraints is sometimes salutary. Worship of Dionysus allows that release to be ritualised and regulated.

Dr Highbrow chose to use Wole Soyinka's translation of the play, noting that it had once been used for a performance at the academy under Banda. It was one of the only works of that playwright not proscribed by his censorship board. Soyinka adapted Euripides to a West African context, and his feel for its universality encouraged us. Our cast was drawn from academy pupils but, to help with the production, Dr Highbrow turned to Felix Sangala.

Mr Sangala had been described to me as 'a man of many parts'. And indeed he was a farmer (as were all able-bodied men), a village headman, a potter, an entrepreneur who ran a rape-oil syndicate, a presence on various local committees and lead singer in the band he had founded.

More controversially, he was also a renowned *fisi* or 'hyena man'.

The *fisi* most commonly helps beget children for husbands who are impotent. But sexual activity is also sometimes ritualised among the Chewa, and, by tradition, certain occasions demand that a woman have intercourse. In the absence of a husband, the *fisi* can be paid by the family to provide this. One such occasion is on attaining widowhood: Sangala might be called upon to sleep with the bereaved on the night of her husband's funeral. And there are various other possible indications – including sometimes prior to a girl's wedding, or at her second menses.

But it was not for any of these parts that we sought out Sangala; rather it was because he was a senior member of the Nyau, the secret society whose members dance *gule wamkulu* – the Great Dance that Dr Highbrow had tried to explain to me on my first night in Malaŵi. In this role, Sangala had developed impressive skills as a mask-maker, and we hoped these would translate into the manufacture of theatrical props for *The Bacchae*.

Sangala was in his late forties, with a short, wiry frame and an untidy grizzled beard. His voice was gentle and hesitant, and he had a warm, playful smile. His eyes were kind but could suddenly glisten with the crazed excitement of the amateur enthusiast. His whole expression had a mercurial quality, suggesting a capacity for mischief. I explained the plot of *The Bacchae*, and he nodded approvingly before asking what masks we would need.

Rehearsals took place after school, in similar conditions to the extra Greek and Latin classes. Sangala attended to assist with costumes and choreography, but his first encounter with the pupils was awkward. Though he had put on his best clothes, he had the unmistakable appearance of a peasant when set beside the children in their smart school uniforms. For their part, they eyed him warily – a visitation from a world some had only recently put behind themselves.

The tension was eased after a few words in the vernacular (technically forbidden at the academy), and then dissolved completely in the riot of donning costumes. Sangala had excelled himself. King Pentheus wore the leopard skin and baboon's tail diadem of an Ngoni chieftain. His mother Agave tinkled with the accoutrements of witchcraft: genets' teeth and fowl bones, feathers and strips of sack-cloth. The king's men brandished clubs and hunting spears; the bacchic revellers metamorphosed into half-beasts with snarling fangs, scabrous manes, horns, tails and snouts. Dionysus was presented as Chimbano, the fearsome bull-crocodile from *gule wamkulu*.

Sangala took charge of the dancing. I had failed completely with this, my fussy efforts at direction resulting only in a cloddish routine that left everyone uninspired. Under Sangala's lead they immediately improvised a dance that was natural, weightless, exultant. Sangala wore the mask of Dionysus and shook a tin-can filled with beans and wedged on a stick. It was a Nyau rattle, and he used it to shake out an ancient rhythm that summoned up instincts which my pupils had kept buried under my direction. On the mountains of Thessaly, scholars and fee-payers, Pentheus and his sisters, princes and peasants, man and beast danced perfectly in step on the stage of Banda's Greek theatre while the moon rose slowly in the failing light.

The actual performances did not quite result in the cultural epiphany we had hoped for. They were well received, especially in the village, where an enormous crowd had gathered. Many families had walked miles for the spectacle, and I had a sense of how seldom anything out of the ordinary was ever made to happen in rural Malaŵi.

It perhaps explained the appetite for witch aeroplanes and other instances of the bizarre.

But the audience's reactions were unpredictable. When Sangala's beasts charged the front seats, the crowd recoiled fearfully, and a few spectators fled in panic. Oddly, the rending and eating of King Pentheus aroused no such horror. It was simulated with 'ration meat' procured from the 'butchery' and mangled in the players' hands. Even when droplets of water were scattered over the audience to mimic spurting blood, the reaction fell short of Aristotelian catharsis – in fact, everyone collapsed into giggles.

The audience kept up a tumultuous wall of chatter, roaring and laughing, so the actors' voices were mostly inaudible. There was no way the action of the play could be followed except as a sort of mime drama. Afterwards a colleague overheard some members discussing the performance: they had clearly enjoyed themselves but were adamant they had witnessed an enactment of Christ's Passion.

As I would shortly discover, the village had little need of Euripides' prescriptions – they had their own. But they had witnessed Dr Highbrow's world and theirs brought together. They had seen both taken seriously, afforded time and respect. It was a start: the gulf had been made slightly smaller, and real effort shown to be expended on something besides subsistence. The poetry did not matter; the contact was everything.

X

THE COMMUNICATION OF THE DEAD

The visceral reaction to Sangala's masked beasts seemed to stem from their resemblance to *gule wamkulu* characters. These had touched a cultural nerve far beyond the reach of even the most compelling of Greek tragedies. When Dr Highbrow had previously tried to explain *gule*, the phenomenon and its terminology bewildered me. Now, however, my curiosity was reignited.

Just as I had been told before, 'They are dead men who come out of the graves to dance for us,' Sangala reaffirmed. I asked if he would show me some *gule*, and he suggested we have a party at his village to celebrate the conclusion of the play. It was possible, though by no means guaranteed, that *gule* might condescend to visit. A date was set, and I agreed to supply Fanta, firewood and a few live goats. Sangala's villagers would brew the maize beer.

As Dr Highbrow reminded me, *gule wamkulu* means 'the Great Dance'. It is a masquerade performed by the Nyau at rites of passage and other occasions of exaltation, sorrow and joy. But it is also a store-house of history and morality, lessons and fables, all identified with particular masks.

Members of the Nyau are initiated through occult rituals. When they don the masks, they undergo metaphysical transformation into ancestral spirits, assuming phantasmagorical form to instruct us. The ancestors are believed to inhabit a world parallel to our own – 'the village on the other side'. Through *gule*, they are able to cross over to the village of the living to impart wisdom and advice. When W.H. Auden and T.S. Eliot spoke of 'the communication of the dead', they had in mind high literature. But it is also a precise definition of *gule*.

At Dr Highbrow's house I had already seen the masks of Chadzunda, an idealised village elder and the father of *gule*; Chipembere, a politicised rhinoceros whose songs subverted the regime in the Banda years; and Kanyoni, who immortalises the spite of a British colonial officer from the 1930s called Henry Kenyon. The masks are heavy, grotesquely fashioned from wood, and boldly painted in red, black and yellow. Chadzunda's expression is broad and gentle, but the face is intricately carved so that countless other tiny *gule* figures appear to crawl from under his skin. Chipembere is distinguished by a mane of banana leaves and exaggerated horns, grossly styled to resemble gigantic phalluses. Kanyoni has the sallow face of the *azungu* with thin, mean lips twisted into a rictus smile beneath a fussy black moustache.

These were only a tiny sample of the pantheon, which is a living, growing thing. Forever added to and adapted, it is potentially infinite, with distinctions blurred between past and present, human and animal, animate and inanimate, abstract and concrete.

The beasts of the forest are all represented: the lion dignifies the installation of chiefs, the elephant mourns at their funerals; the jackal and python confer potency; a mischievous squirrel soothes domestic strife. Even pubic lice are acknowledged.

The minibus also dances, censuring corruption; the whirlwind warns against discord; the bicycle in one village celebrates innovation, in another deplores it.

Big Men, native and foreign, historical and contemporary abound: Banda has multiple instantiations, some good, some evil. President Bingu, Pope John Paul II, King Edward VII and our late Queen Elizabeth all dance together with the incarnations of Peace and Propriety, Envy, Slander and Unrest. Dr Highbrow once saw a jiggling worm-like figure who was explained as the minatory wagging finger of a severe local trader.

Many dancers evoke the world of nightmare: the stumps of leprosy are simulated with dirty sacking bound tight around face, hands and feet; HIV by a naked figure who torches his pubic hair with flaming brands. Various characters with obscene names educate young girls in menstrual hygiene. One is besmirched with filth; his lips and eyelids are retracted with wires to suggest symptoms of *mdulo*, a wasting disease believed to be contracted by breach of sexual taboo.

What intrigued me most was the discovery that *gule* had found a bizarre reflex in the early years of Kamuzu Academy. Samson Kambalu is today aprofessor of contemporary art at Oxford, and the sculptor of Trafalgar Square's new statue of John Chilembwe. He was educated at the academy, but before he arrived as a teenager in the 1980s, he had already been initiated into the Nyau. His memoir, *The Jive Talker*, describes dormitories rife with strange rituals, in which the prefects assumed characters that echoed the world of *gule* but were inspired by the academy's curriculum.

There were Dionysus and Diogenes, Orpheus and Heraclitus, Pliny and Caligula, Roman Nose and The Twelve Caesars. But other features of the school besides Classics had clearly impressed themselves on the boys: Rommel and

Richelieu were incarnated, as were Sit Down Don't Argue and Keep Off the Grass. One character gleefully identified himself as The Book of Revelation and the Monsters Therein. Kambalu became Sisero, and this remained his *gule* character outside school when he rejoined the Nyau of his home district. He describes how, on one occasion, Sisero upbraided a party of bumptious evangelical missionaries with his oratory, urging them to 'f--- off' in Latin.

At that time many pupils had never before left their villages, let alone engaged with the study of Greece and Rome. And so they adapted their own ways of coping with the strange world that now confronted them. In *gule* they possessed a lifeline to what they had left behind. As their old identity was buffeted by an alien culture, village tradition became their ballast, keeping them upright amid the upheaval.

I knew little of what went on in the boarding houses after dusk, but I suspect that this tradition of pseudo-*gule* might have vanished from the academy by the time I got there. In the village, however, *gule* was very much alive.

XI

THE GREAT DANCE

I drove out with Dr Highbrow to Sangala's village. It was winter – a time of conviviality in Malaŵi, when the harvest is in and there is little work to be done in the bare fields. We passed a large cattle farm where the land opened out wide and flat beneath a pink sun hovering just above the horizon. It was briefly clouded over by a dense flock of egrets that we disturbed from a spinney of trees. The road dipped down beside a dry riverbed, and we entered a large depression previously invisible from view. We managed to negotiate a route around a broken culvert, and were then edging down tiny lanes, banked with the last of the year's wild flowers.

Drawing closer, we passed more and more parties of villagers walking in the same direction. They waved and shouted excitedly and then, at the edge of Sangala's village, gathered in a throng around our vehicle. For the last few hundred yards, they trotted beside us, tugging and hammering high-spiritedly at the windows and body-work.

When we arrived, the crowd parted as Sangala stepped forward at the head of a reception committee. There followed ritualised welcomes from his wife and family, other elders, local chiefs. Then Sangala asked us, with a coy smile, if we wanted to meet the man with three wives. We said we would be delighted, and Sangala beamed. He took us to a hut set apart from the rest, and introduced us to a bashful but good-looking man in middle age who bowed as we shook hands.

'This,' Sangala announced, 'is the man with three wives.'

We exchanged pleasantries for a time, until at length I asked if we might meet the wives. There followed a slightly tense consultation with Sangala, after which the man called inside the hut, and three dignified young women stepped out, gracefully attired in *chitenjes*, colourful lengths of cloth worn as a dress. They kept their eyes lowered but smiled slightly coquettishly as they curtsied before us, one by one.

'I built this house with my own hands,' declared the man with three wives, gesturing towards the mud-brick structure, which had clearly been constructed with care and looked after. The walls were smoothly daubed, the thatch tightly woven. Unlike so many roofs in Malaŵi, this one looked as if it might actually repel rain. Glowing marigolds had been planted in front of the *khonde*, from which you could enjoy a fine view over distant hills. The whole was shielded from the rest of the community by a bank of sedge grass shimmering iridescent in the breeze. We remarked that it was a very good house, and the man blushed with gratification.

'I built this house with my own hands,' he repeated.

We thanked him and exchanged further courtesies before being led back to the centre of the village.

'What is his religion, Mr Sangala?' I asked. I was not being prudish: it was a question that was asked almost routinely in Malaŵi.

Sangala thought for a while and then answered cautiously: 'That one, he is not a church-goer.'

A large clearing had been prepared beside the village: debris had been removed, the earth stamped flat, the surface fastidiously swept. A fire was being lit at its centre. A row of chairs had been laid out, among them even an armchair in worn crimson velvet that had been hauled a considerable distance to its position of honour beneath a mango tree. Dr Highbrow was invited to occupy this seat, and we took our places beside him.

There were about ten huts ringed with fruit trees and, beyond them, rows of onions and ground-nuts springing up in small patches of cleared earth amid the scrub. The land declined towards a marsh dense with foliage. In the distance, there were only empty plains as far as the dark forests around Chipata Mountain thirty miles away.

Sangala's village had moved three times in almost as many years owing to squabbles over land rights. Everything in the area belonged to two or three farmers, who periodically evicted Sangala, an illegal squatter. On the last occasion, the huts had been razed with tractors and the fields sowed with lime. Sangala had managed to salvage his tin roof from the destruction before he and the other men of the village were thrown into Kasungu prison. They had been let out before the next growing season and re-established themselves at the site we were now visiting. Sangala had rebuilt his hut, and his tin roof (the only one in the village) sheltered him once more.

Sangala's good cheer was irrepressible, even in the face of eviction; his people clung to him throughout these upheavals. He was also receptive to strangers, and introduced us to a newcomer in his village – a man originally from Dedza, almost 150 miles away, who had spent months wandering from misfortune. He was a good musician, and Sangala offered him shelter on the strength of this. A connoisseur of music and song, Sangala needed players for his band. Three of these musicians now took up position by the fire and played elegantly on guitars improvised from refuse.

Now and then, Sangala and his sons sang to their accompaniment. The lyrics were Sangala's own and related an incomprehensible love story. There was then an old praise song about Kamuzu Banda, a ballad of the village's tribulations and a paean celebrating the beneficence of Dr Highbrow, who had paid for and supervised the construction of the nearest school. I recognised words with which my colleague's vehicle had been hailed by passers-by on the journey over. Dr Highbrow was looking at the ground shyly.

The sun had still not quite set, but both the moon and the evening star were already high in a sky of dark blue. The crowd was enormous, and the chatter began to make the warm-up act inaudible. Several drums were beating slowly, and the air was heavy with yeast from the vast plastic vats of thick maize beer which the wives were stirring with rough sticks. In the clearing, the girls received instructions while the old women began to dance slowly in rings. Some were very aged, but all swayed to the same ponderous rhythm as they stomped deliberately round the fire, slowly clapping their hands. They described circles within circles, tilting back their heads to send up peals of laughter and songs of contentment into the rotating firmament.

I found myself thinking back to a scene from Lucretius, who shied away from the harsh cosmopolitanism of Ancient Rome and turned instead to prehistory and the world's primordial origins. In his poem *On the Nature of the Universe*, he imagined the discovery of music by early man. Enraptured by the call of birds and nature's beauty, he felt compelled to express his joy first in movement and then in song, traipsing carelessly through woods and flowers before falling into step and learning dance.

The circles grew larger, and the elders were joined and replaced by younger women as the drumming quickened.

They were gyrating rapidly now, and the onlookers whooped with delight from the sides of the clearing. Some of the younger girls held back from the fray but were increasingly teased for their recalcitrance: there was much giggling and suggestive thrusting of hips in their direction. Eventually, they were all encouraged to step forward and copy the others. Those that thrust their hips most vigorously were singled out and applauded for their displays of youthful fecundity.

We remained seated, shivering slightly – when the sun sets at this time of year, the temperature drops precipitously. The old men remained beside us, but Sangala was nowhere to be seen. The beer was being liberally distributed: it was sour and lumpy, with the consistency of thin porridge. It was still a little warm from fermentation and did seem to ward off the chill settling on us as the darkness deepened. Soon the only light came from the fire, moon and stars. The figures hurtling around us became blurred as they throbbed ever faster.

Just as the movements were taking on a dull, rhythmic conformity, the crowd froze suddenly and a few squeals were uttered. They had sensed something to which we were oblivious, but the drumming never ceased, and the dancing was quickly resumed. This happened two or three times before I at last detected the sound of a rattle, quiet but close at hand.

Then with screams of excitement, the crowd was violently sundered as a warthog in a sisal kilt leapt into the clearing, shaking a tin can filled with beans, like the one that had appeared at the Greek play. The warthog used this to beckon onto the stage Chadzunda, hobbling and bent double over a crooked stick. He limped feebly but rhythmically around the clearing, while the crowd laughed with delighted approval. His mask, less elaborate than the one I had seen in Dr Highbrow's house, was still recognisable as an old man with a kindly face, scored with white-on-black carving, like an early Attic vase. He was clad in strips of fertiliser sacking woven into an elaborate 'tatter suit' of fluttering multi-coloured strands that puffed up like a bush as he moved. At first he gave a faultless performance of elderly frailty, but then he straightened himself and leapt high in the air before prancing acrobatically to symbolise vigour concealed in old age.

He was joined presently by his wife, Mariya, fair-faced and smiling, bedecked with bangles and beads, and with a halo of banana leaves about her head. They danced together in dignified and commodious union, while the women sang of the joys of happy matrimony. When their time was up, the warthog rattled them off the stage and the women's dances resumed.

At these events, the Nyau operate from a temporary secret camp set apart from the village and known as the *dambwe*. It is traditionally located at a graveyard, and the dancers are supposed to emerge, undead, from the tombs. Graveyards are generally given a wide berth in Malaŵi, and, if the Nyau are present, trespassers can be repelled ferociously.

The *dambwe* on this occasion seemed to be down in the marshy depression, and it was from there that the warthog returned, this time leading in Makanja, a figure clad in glorious patchwork and swaying on stilts. The agility was extraordinary: a jute helmet obscured his view, so it was only by the lead of the rattle that he knew where to step. He skipped furiously around the flames, occasionally even leaping but still landing squarely. His lesson was how the mighty fall: periodically he would trip on a maize cob left at his feet by the warthog. But after staggering precariously, he would then thrust himself upright before dancing on to cheers and raucous laughter.

When Makanja returned to the *dambwe*, there was a further interval during which the women formed ever more complicated intersecting rings, weaving in and out among each other. Every woman for miles around must have been dancing when at last the warthog reappeared. But this time there was something menacing in his movements, and the women seemed fretful and excited.

Suddenly, they erupted in screams of terror as the warthog beckoned in Chimbano, striding slowly but heavily like a cinema dinosaur. He was horrifying: a mutant crocodile-bull with a monstrous red face beset with jagged teeth. But it was his wooden snout that was most appalling: it was grossly protuberant and carved to resemble male and female sex organs in coition. Chimbano began to rush the throng of women, who recoiled in waves from his advances. He would then himself retire before charging again. Soon, he and the dancers were engaged in a throbbing *pas de deux*: the women moved back and forth in response to his feints and withdrawals, faster and faster until they all seemed to thrust together as one. Intermittently, though, Chimbano would overtake the crowd and snatch a girl from it, pressing her briefly to his horrible face before tossing her back. The warthog now brandished an enormous wooden phallus, which he threateningly urged the girls to touch. He sang a bawdy song, explained to me as a lesson in the importance of wiping clean your husband's penis after he ejaculates.

The drumming reached a frenzy, beating faster than you believed possible, so that it dissolved into a wall of white noise to which the dancers thrust their hips with the speed and force of piston engines. The beer was making me feel giddy and slightly sick. Half-remembered words of the Roman playwright Terence rang in my head: '*nihil humani alienum mihi puto.*' I must consider nothing human as alien to me.

This was the domain of Dionysus: 'the liquid fire in the grape, the sap thrusting in a young tree, the blood pounding in the veins of a young animal, all the mysterious and uncontrollable tides that ebb and flow in the life of nature', as an editor of *The Bacchae*, E.R. Dodds, had once written, no doubt in a dusty, book-lined Oxford study.

And then memory led me back to Oxford. Or rather to a remote field on a country estate outside the city, owned by the family of a fellow student. We had been taken there by bus on a deliberately circuitous route to obscure the location. Everyone was dressed in a perversion of formal wear: ball-gowns and bondage gear; white tie and Bullingdon tails with animal-head masks; military dress coats and fish-net stockings. The field was pumped with the deafening thud of techno music that reached a pitch somewhere between a scream and an explosion as the crowd pulsated in a stupor of champagne and amphetamines. Figures slipped (or were dragged?) away from the main frenzy of activity. Slinking half-naked into bushes, bodies revealed their whereabouts by convulsive animal movements, felt more than seen in the undergrowth.

Dr Highbrow shook me from my stupor: 'Would you agree it is probably time for us to leave? I think we have seen enough.' We crept off, our parting barely noticed by our distracted hosts. As we were negotiating the track from the village, a couple of *lende* figures darted across our path. They were naked and smeared in mud, with black fabric tightly bound around their heads and only narrow slits for eyes. They wielded sticks and panga knives and moved fast and judderingly, like figures caught in strobe lighting. In a second they were gone. *Lende* enforce the rule of the Nyau – on each other and hapless villagers who cross their path. 'I think we have seen enough,' repeated Dr Highbrow.

For some time afterwards, I did not know how to reckon with the mixture of brutality and exuberance I had seen. At Oxford, the ecstasy had been hollow amusement, the product of ennui. We could not reaffirm our connection with each other or with the place, because we didn't know where we were; in the morning, we were bussed back to resume our discrete, atomised existences. It had been a brief excursion from reality, safe, meaningless and, above all, sterile.

For Sangala's villagers, the frenzied animalism expressed their indomitable will to survive. They were claiming and consecrating that place as their own; the place where, together, they would live and die, endure and multiply. The village children had been exposed to graphic and vigorous demonstrations of the facts of life. But unlike the barren pornography their Western peers might have watched, this was a celebration of fertility. As I would soon see for myself, the threat of death hung heavy and constant over their world. It could only be defied with a vitality so strong it knew violence.

A few years later, I was re-reading T.S. Eliot's 'East Coker' and its description of an English village dance in rural Somerset. It is the twentieth century, but the dancers divest their modernity to reveal a coarse inner core that is ancient and true. I was assailed with the full force of *déjà vu* as the poem transported me back to Sangala's village:

> [. . .] Round and round the fire
> Leaping through the flames, or joined in circles,
> Rustically solemn or in rustic laughter
> Lifting heavy feet in clumsy shoes,

> Earth feet, loam feet, lifted in country mirth,
> Mirth of those long since under earth,
> Nourishing the corn. Keeping time,
> Keeping the rhythm in their dancing
> As in their living the living seasons
> The time of the seasons and the constellations,
> The time of milking and the time of harvest,
> The time of the coupling of man and woman,
> And that of beasts. Feet rising and falling.
> Eating and drinking. Dung and death.

I had come to regard the Modernist poets, like Eliot, with growing sympathy. The strangeness of Malaŵian society made me appreciate their struggle to elucidate the past, even its obscurest ritual, for our bewildered present. I would soon discover Malaŵi had its own recent poetic tradition that attempted the same thing.

In 'East Coker', the gentility of contemporary life is shattered by an eruption of the primitive, forcing us to acknowledge man as dying animal, part of the surrounding earth in its cycle of decay and procreation. There is no escape from the ugliness of 'dung and death', but there is also the mirth of the Great Dance – the dance of rapturous, enduring humanity.

XII

DEATH

&

TRANSFIGURATION

Back on the tobacco farm, it emerged that Lysard Moyo's daughter had been ill for some time. I had heard nothing of this until one day he appealed to me for transport to the hospital. He had wanted to contact me a few days before but the cell-phone I had given him was out of battery. To charge it, he had had to walk ten miles to Wimbe and, when he got there, a long power cut had just begun. When power was restored, he had to pay and wait for the phone to be charged, staying overnight in an acquaintance's goat pen. He then had to walk back.

By the time I got to his house, after he called me, his daughter was drifting in and out of consciousness. I had never set eyes on her before and had not in fact known of her existence. She had apparently been confined to the hut for many days.

Lysard Moyo and his sons lifted her into the back of the Land Rover. She was about my age and strikingly beautiful. She looked as if she were sleeping peacefully, but when she opened her eyes for a moment, they were livid with jaundice. Then she vomited a pint or more of fresh red blood.

It was about a half-hour drive to the hospital down sludgy dirt roads that were here and there turning to quagmire. She was unconscious for the journey but started vomiting blood again almost as soon as she was moved from the vehicle. There was no doctor employed by the hospital, but she was seen by a clinical officer with some experience. He palpated her abdomen and remarked on her massively enlarged spleen. He gave her some fluids and prepared to take blood samples from the whole family in case one turned out to be a matching donor for a transfusion. This might help, he explained, but the girl was fading fast, and he doubted there was much he could do. She was in liver failure – perhaps secondary to Hepatitis B, he suspected.

As he was talking, she woke again and, in an unexpected display of strength, pushed herself up off the bed to stare at us for a moment. Then she vomited even more profusely before sinking back drenched in her own blood. She passed away about a minute later.

The clinical officer offered his condolences and moved on to his next patient. At that moment there rose from Lysard Moyo a groan that grew louder and louder until, in that confined space, it might have been the sound of the earth rending in two. It went on and on so that it felt like it would never cease. And when it did finally abate, Lysard Moyo paused only for a second to catch his breath before starting again. He fell to his knees, tore at his face and hair with his hands, touched his forehead to the floor and beat it with his massive rough fists. The rest of the family joined in the lament, filling the room with the sound of agony. I looked around to see the other patients staring fearfully at us. They had seen everything.

We took her body back to the farm, and Lysard Moyo later buried her at the foot of an acacia tree on the edge of his maize patch. I did not know the girl and was unsure about attending the funeral. But, in the event, Lysard Moyo's phone battery had died again so the dilemma did not arise. I later saw her grave and thought of the small plot of earth now enfolding her. Those few acres of land had been her entire life. Its soil had brought forth every meal she had ever eaten, the mud-bricks and straw that had sheltered her, even the bed on which she had slept. And now 'the life-giving earth that holds fast even him that is strong' had reclaimed her. It was as if her being, like the autochthonous creatures of Ancient Greece, had never been separate from it.

When I later started working in UK hospitals, I became aware of how tidily death is managed in the West. Even when not well planned, it is usually well hidden: an alarm sounds, clinicians gather, any commotion takes place behind drawn curtains.

In Malaŵi, death seemed omnipresent. Every village had its coffin workshop, advertised by a hand-painted sign: 'Super Coffins', 'Comfort Coffins', 'Heaven Bound Coffins', even 'Energy Coffins' and, most poignantly, 'Family Coffins'. Even in the less than Arcadian world of the academy, death kept his court. I first witnessed this when the carpenter left my house cheerfully one evening but failed to appear for work the next day. After that, I became more alert to the macabre quality of the staff noticeboard which, Dr Highbrow observed, only ever featured death notices and sausage advertisements. (The sausages were manufactured and sold by various colleagues as a way to supplement their incomes.)

One memorable afternoon, as we sipped gin and tonics at the staff club during a rainstorm, we were interrupted by squeals from a trio of children gathered outside at the edge of the swimming pool. They were cooing and pointing at a corpse floating face down in the water. Though it was later identified as the cook of a local farmer, explanations for its presence there were not entirely satisfying.

A few pupils passed away almost every year, and the names of the deceased would be read out during assembly. They were lost to road accidents, malaria, HIV and a host of other diseases that would mostly have been treatable elsewhere.

Grace, a popular girl who was also one of my more conscientious pupils, died of malaria during term-time, and her class was shaken. Her best friend dedicated her music-exam recital to her, singing 'What Is Life?' from Gluck's *Orpheus and Eurydice*. The audience, who usually babbled and fidgeted intolerably at any other school concert, listened with solemn attention.

She was accompanied on the piano by Mr Leonard Chisomo, the head of music. He was a complicated man who had intended to be ordained as a priest but had been driven from his seminary in disgrace. This had taken place over a decade before but clearly continued to sting. He would protest his innocence to anyone who would listen, solemnly explaining how he had one night been caught *leaving* the dormitories of an adjacent women's college. His subsequent expulsion had been a gross injustice as the rules were quite clear: they only prohibited *entering* the dormitories, and of this his accusers had had no proof. His listeners often found the story amusing, and Mr Chisomo would stare at his feet and shake his head with a half-smile of exasperation.

He was well read, and the first time I met him he had just returned from an ascent of Mount Mulanje, where he had retreated to read *Northanger Abbey* in seclusion. He also helped with teaching Latin from time to time, having studied this during his short-lived preparation for the priesthood. But it was as director of music that he advertised himself most prominently. He was said to be working on an opera and certainly had an exhibitionist streak that delighted in the pomp and fanfare of official visits and Founder's Day. On these occasions, he would assemble large and torturous combinations of electronic instruments that could render even famous works unrecognisable. Ambassadors sometimes attended to give out the prizes and would have to grimace as their national anthems were duly mutilated. It felt as though Malaŵians possessed an extraordinary, almost innate musicality, that would be discarded when electricity was available.

Mr Chisomo really did appreciate music, though, and was capable of performing it to a very high standard. I remember walking past his classroom late one evening, drawn by the sound of a lonely piano. He was playing alone in the darkness, and I recognised the aroma of *chamba* smoke and the unexpected notes of Hindemith drifting through the window. He then moved on to a Bach Prelude, and I listened in secret, gazing up at the constellations. The gentle but resolute orderliness amid complexity was soothing at the end of that sorrowful term.

In the village, the choir of Saint Mary's Outstation, just outside the academy, gathers in the open to rehearse at close of day. The singers drift in from the fields, the women bearing and balancing great loads on their heads, the men still clutching hoes. The fainting sun forms long shadows as they take their places on rough benches beneath a baobab.

The choirmaster is a serious man and welcomes our interest without obsequiousness. At the summons of his hands, the choir surges as if with one voice, an enormous, miraculous sound in that recently silent and empty place. Their synchronisation is perfect, so the hostile world seems suddenly confronted by a warm but defiant wall of music.

A single hand drum and a few maracas are their only accompaniment and add a vigorous, march-like quality. The melodies perhaps owe something to European hymns, but the rhythms and harmonies are purely African and exquisitely complicated. Faces strain with concentration, as if to restrain emotion that might otherwise explode.

Amid so much poverty, it can be easy for outsiders to grow accustomed to shoddiness, to the feeling that excellence in anything must always remain out of reach. The choir's music is exhilarating not only for its intricate beauty but also for the self-respect and spirit of perfectionism on display. It is as though nothing could be more important than those richly affirmative songs through which, despite everything, joy is proclaimed and thanks given for all the gifts of the earth.

PART TWO
NGWAZI

XIII

THE WANDERER

In this same village of Mtunthama, a hundred years before, the young Hastings Kamuzu Banda attended a small Scottish missionary school where he was taught basic literacy and numeracy. But his intelligence demanded more, and further education could only be found elsewhere. In about 1915, still a teenager, he left home, taking with him a knife, a spear, a club, some string, three shillings he had saved and food for a few days only. He said goodbye to his parents, whom he would never see again, and set his sights on the Lovedale Missionary Institute, 1,500 miles away in South Africa. It was reputed to offer the best education available to black students anywhere on the continent, and even taught Latin and Greek. But Banda got waylaid.

After wandering through Portuguese Mozambique, he found his way to a hospital in Rhodesia, where he swept floors but also impressed the doctor, who invited him to observe his clinics and procedures – experiences which, Banda said, stirred his earliest interest in medicine. After a year or two, he set off again and this time reached Johannesburg.

He travelled largely on foot, begging food and shelter along the way and encountering, for the most part, only kindness and generosity. Now, in the great urban melting pot, he was struck by the contrast: 'There was no feeling of the Africa I knew. All of the tradition and culture was gone and in its place was crime and evil. I felt great sadness at how far African people had fallen.'

Banda never made it to Lovedale. Far from it – he stayed on the Rand and toiled in the mines. He eventually found less brutal work as a clerk, and this might well have been the pinnacle of his career – but he was about to achieve something miraculous. He had continued to attend school whenever he could, and his talents were eventually recognised. Through church networks, he won sponsorship to study in America.

In 1925 he sailed from South Africa to England and on to New York. He enrolled at Wilberforce Academy in Ohio to study a broad programme of English, mathematics, literature and Classics. After this, he took a degree in history and dabbled in anthropology at the universities of Chicago and Indiana. Finally he switched to medicine, qualifying in 1937 from Meharry, Tennessee. He still had no money of his own and was supported by a small but close-knit community of African émigrés, generally associated through their churches.

Banda's experiences in America were complicated. Besides acquiring a profession, he was immersing himself delightedly in the cultural riches of Western civilisation. At the same time, he reached back to his own heritage with an exile's heightened sense of identity. He collaborated with several American academics on their ethnographic projects and welcomed their interest and encouragement to reminisce about the world he had left behind. 'It cured me of my tendency to be ashamed of my past,' he later confessed.

But he was not only far from home. He was a black man living in America during the era of segregation and Jim Crow laws. He was surprised to find himself treated politely enough by white people but realised this was because he was African (rather than a Black American) and thus a beneficiary of weird exemptions from the prevailing racism. He could not fail to witness the mistreatment of other black people, nor to absorb the atmosphere of racial menace and contempt. In Nashville he chanced upon a lynching and watched, unmolested but helpless, as the Ku Klux Klan slung their battered victim from a tree to hang.

He spent over a decade in America and had to adapt to what he found. His inspiration was a Black American surgeon, Walter Bailey, who welcomed him to his home and practice during university vacations. Banda noticed that Bailey seemed to stand above prejudice and was sought after by patients both black and white, on account of his professional reputation: 'It was a very good lesson to me,' Banda noted, 'to always be the best. The best has no barriers, racial or otherwise.' It was an elitist and individualistic response: useless to other victims, it was Banda's way of coping with his peculiar circumstances.

His plan had been to qualify as a doctor and then return home to serve his own people. But his degree was not valid for work outside America. So now, aged almost forty, he sailed to Britain for further medical studies, securing sponsorship from the imperial government in Nyasaland and the Church of Scotland.

The contrast with segregated America astonished Banda. Until this point, he had cut a shy, retiring figure: 'He was very smart but just had nothing to say,' was the judgement of one Chicago landlady. In Britain he relaxed, began to open up, became gregarious, even. He had found a correspondent in Chief Mwase back in Malaŵi, and wrote excitedly about his experiences. He had never been mistreated in America, he insisted. But it was nothing like Britain, where he now associated freely with Europeans, meeting and sitting beside them in church, restaurants, theatres, picture-houses. Mwase did not believe Banda until he visited him in London a few years later. The chief then wrote a poignant letter back to his family: 'I did not think a European could be as kind and respectful to an African as the letters suggested. But I can see now that Dr Banda was right.'

It was in Scotland that he received the warmest welcome. Raised a Presbyterian, his sensibilities were initially horrified by the Scots' enthusiasm for pubs and dance-halls, but Banda overcame this when he found himself becoming something of a local celebrity in Edinburgh. The city was awash with retired missionaries and old Africa hands, many of whom were acquainted even with his village in Kasungu. When he first encountered them, he broke down in tears as they reminisced about the places they had in common. He was adopted by this circle and formed several lifelong friendships. They received him into their houses, supported his work and studies, took him in to convalesce after he needed surgery for appendicitis.

He was beginning his own medical practice around this time, having refused military service in World War Two on conscientious grounds. He discovered an affinity with the impoverished patients of Leith, the poor quarter of the city where he was assigned. But he was equally comfortable playing bridge in the Edinburgh Student Union. Still, there were limits to his acceptance: he is said to have courted three young women but secured the hand of none. The details are murky, but, in at least one case, marriage was opposed by the girl's family because he was black. Decades later it was reported that she never married, and that Banda had been the love of her life.

Scotland furnished him with almost a surrogate identity, but he still spoke of feeling homesick even after many decades in the West. In 1940 he was ordained as an Elder of the Kirk of Scotland at the Guthrie Memorial Church on Edinburgh's Easter Road. The investiture, he said, 'felt like a homecoming': 'I was surrounded by many, many friends, friends who knew my family in Kasungu, my sisters, my uncles. Because they were present, I felt that my own family was present.'

After four years, medical duties took Banda to Liverpool then Tyneside, where he tended burns victims during the Blitz. He was remembered decades later for his kindness: he frequently waived medical fees and even helped a number of his poorest patients with their rent. At the end of the war, he relocated to London, selecting Harlesden for his GP surgery because he was struck by the peculiar friendliness of the residents as he wandered one day among their bombed-out houses. For almost ten years he commuted from Willesden Green in his black Austin, greeted on arrival by a waiting-room of patients who honoured him by standing to their feet as he entered.

Now in his fifties, Banda began to drift from medicine into politics. Indeed, the Nyasaland government noted his anti-colonial activities and contrived obstacles to prevent him from starting a practice there. This only intensified his intrigues in London, where he had to buy a bigger house to accommodate the comings and goings of African nationalists and their sympathisers. Nkrumah, Kenyatta, Nyerere, Labour MPs and half the Fabian Society wandered in and out of his drawing room, stoking discontent. By virtue of his age and experience, Banda was already the elder statesman among Africa's fledgling leaders.

His central preoccupation at this time was the British effort to disembarrass itself of Nyasaland and the Rhodesias, and to recreate these possessions as a single colossal territory: the Federation of Central Africa. It was to be an independent state but one ultimately led by a white minority government. Promises were extended to the Africans, but history has condemned the Federation as a greedy ploy to combine the natural resources of Northern Rhodesia (now Zambia) with the manpower of Nyasaland, all under the direction of the white overlords of Southern Rhodesia (now Zimbabwe), who would rule unencumbered by the moderating influence of the Colonial Office in London.

Opposition to this was the basis of Banda's campaign for independence, and he became the focal point for a network of dissidents. These prepared the ground for his return so that when at last he went home, a tumultuous crowd had assembled to welcome him off the plane. He later described how he scanned the sea of faces, repeatedly deceiving himself that he recognised that of his mother. But it was 1958, he had been away for over forty years, and his parents were both dead.

There was a lot of wrangling as black Nyasaland activists vied with the white Rhodesians, and Her Majesty's Government struggled wearily to arbitrate. This was Banda's hour of triumph: he toured the country relentlessly, stirring up resistance to the Federation. He discovered a gift for portentous oratory and commanded bigger and bigger audiences, whom he could whip into a frenzy with his freedom cry of '*Kwacha!*' – 'Dawn!'

There were flashes of violence; Banda was imprisoned for just over a year; thirty-three people were killed when troops fired on a rioting mob at Nkhata Bay. But for the most part, Banda avowed peaceful means, soon emerging, even in the eyes of the colonial government, as the worthiest and most qualified man to take over power. Britain was trying to discard African possessions with the minimum possible hassle. The Rhodesians' vision of Federation was rejected, and Nyasaland gained independence in 1964. Banda became her first president, renamed the country Malaŵi, and formed a lifelong friendship with the outgoing British governor.

XIV

THE GREAT DICTATOR

Back in the abandoned palace, Dr Highbrow and I evoked biography from trinkets and bibelots of curious provenance. An antique Levantine jar was the gift of the people of Israel, a Roman gold coin that of the Italians. A silver Tiffany cigar box was inscribed with best wishes from Lyndon Johnson yet was set beside souvenir kitsch from the Tower of London, a tea tray adorned with the faces of the Windsors and a complimentary paperweight from the Republic of Venda – one of the South African 'Bantustans'.

In filing cases we found plans, projects and proposals – for railway redevelopment, Kamuzu Academy, Lonrho estates – and a hare-brained scheme for a herbal cure for leprosy, advanced by a German quack physician. Dossier folders yielded the blueprints for Lilongwe, the new capital city built *ex nihilo* in 1971. We spread it out on the purple snakeskin writing set from Asprey and pored over it. With lion skins at our feet, it was easy to conjure a giddy atmosphere of megalomania.

Banda began dispensing with democracy early on. There had been a flash of opposition just after independence and, for a moment, it looked like the venerable doctor might be toppled by a cabal of 'Young Turks' in his own cabinet. A friend of mine was present as a journalist in the Malaŵi parliament when they assailed Banda. Unperturbed, he rose and denounced them – quietly, coldly and with a calm that suggested diabolical confidence. Within two years, all his opponents (much of Malaŵi's youthful talent) were in exile or prison. Banda was unapologetic: if the country really needed qualified administrators, the British would just have to stay on as employees of the new state. He won elections in 1966 as the only candidate. When his first five-year term was up, parliament (which consisted of one party only) voted him President for Life. Later it would confer on him his preferred title, 'Ngwazi' – an ancient honorific variously translated as 'conqueror', 'lion' or 'chief of chiefs'. To others, he was 'one-man Banda'.

His style became more defined. He favoured Savile Row suits, with a starched white handkerchief in the top pocket, a red carnation in the button-hole. Out and about, he wore a Burberry mackintosh and carried a cane. There were hats for every occasion, but his most iconic was the Homburg made famous by Anthony Eden. An officer of the Malaŵi Defence Force held a parasol over Banda's head as he walked, and the president assumed the use of a fly-whisk, a symbol of royalty since the age of the pharaohs.

His first of these was inlaid with ivory and silver, a gift from Jomo Kenyatta, who paid him an official visit soon after independence. But Banda quickly fell out with his peers across the continent because of his relations with South Africa and Portugal. At a time when every other black African government was united in their denunciation of the apartheid state and the last European power in Africa, Banda adopted a conciliatory approach. For the South Africans in particular, this was diplomatic gold dust, and they lavished money on Banda's regime – including the funds for his new capital. In 1970 Banda received South Africa's prime minister John Vorster in Malaŵi and paid an official visit to the Republic the following year. He was bitterly reviled at the Organisation for African Unity, while the South Africans gave him a 21-gun salute.

Banda's pragmatic justifications recalled his response to segregation in America. When he visited Stellenbosch, he was received by huge crowds of different races. It was, he insisted, symbolically and psychologically important for *all* South Africans to witness a black man cheered by whites. Neither rhetoric nor violence would bring down the colour bar, he argued. Instead there should be constructive dialogue. In the library, we found an album containing photos of this trip: of Banda and his companion, Cecilia Kadzamira, relaxing at a picnic with President and Mrs Fouché, all smiling genially over tea at Groote Schuur.

Kadzamira was a nurse employed by Banda when he first returned to Malaŵi. Forty years his junior, she became his secretary, confidante, carer and constant companion for the rest of his life. Beyond this, their relationship was never defined; they did not marry and had no offspring. Early on, Kadzamira acquired the ambiguous title, 'Official Government Hostess', which was later formally upgraded to 'Mother of the Nation' or 'Mama'. In this capacity she welcomed the Queen of England and the Emperor of Ethiopia, but her influence began to extend beyond matters of protocol.

At first this seemed harmless: when she took umbrage at the words of the Simon and Garfunkel song 'Cecilia', it was duly banned. But the atmosphere grew slowly more sinister. Her uncle rose high in office and gained a reputation as the government's hatchet man. Political opponents had a convenient habit of disappearing: when they were not incarcerated or hanged for treason, fatal accidents seemed to befall them with marked frequency.

Banda had become very rich. His company, Press Holdings, acquired vast tracts of land and became a conglomerate with diverse interests. Malaŵi was run as a command economy on almost mercantilist lines – a system that actually worked well in the early part of his rule. But it meant the country's resources could be summoned for whatever purpose Banda desired. On tour, he was most famously seen standing in the back of an open-top Land Rover, though a cherry-pink Rolls-Royce was soon added to the cortège. Palaces multiplied. In a back room of Banda's library, we found a box filled with packing foam. Rummaging brought forth the brochure of a manufacturer of private jets, a tarnished Mappin & Webb tea service and a wodge of Laura Ashley sample fabrics. On the wall, a gold Jaeger-LeCoultre clock was cracked and in need of winding.

Banda always made much of avoiding debt as a psychological imperative for a developing nation. Impressively, he had balanced the books soon after independence, and kept things that way for most of his rule. But steely prudence turned into geriatric rigidity. Malaŵi could not afford to coast along: by the 1980s, its population had almost quadrupled since independence, without corresponding economic growth. Public services had once been estimable by the standards of such a poor country. Now they began to fall apart.

As Banda grew older, access to him became increasingly regulated by Mama and her clique. Banda still went on tours of inspection but, in his infirmity, could not or would not look beyond the Potemkin farms, schools and hospitals rigged by devious ministers. The prosperity of earlier years evanesced, AIDS was rampant and, in 1992, the country experienced its first famine since independence. Shortly afterwards, Banda, then in his nineties, became unwell and had to undergo brain surgery abroad. He returned almost completely deaf. People had to address him through a microphone connected to a pair of large headphones. Caroline Alexander, an American Classicist, described talking into this as 'like speaking directly to [Banda's] brain'.

By the end, power was being jostled between rival court factions in an atmosphere of intrigue and paranoia. There had always been a vicious side to the regime but also an odd countervailing current of rectitude. Dictatorship was mostly tolerated as a fair price for order and functionality. Now, however, the brutality escalated, and the victims were many. *Lettres de cachet* circulated, often bearing only clumsily forged versions of Banda's signature. In greater and greater numbers, poets and politicians, teachers, doctors and lawyers fell foul of the hypersensitive regime and were driven to exile, imprisoned or murdered. Meanwhile, the people were bullied by a volatile party youth wing, and corruption at all levels became normalised.

There was never the total dysfunctionality of Tanzania, the chronic shortages of Zambia, the ruination of Zimbabwe or the holocausts of Mozambique, Uganda, Zaïre. But there was cruelty and injustice. How much is directly attributable to Banda is contested. His supporters insist the wickedness emanated from those around him who took advantage of his age and decrepitude. But Banda seemed sometimes to take a malicious relish in bringing retribution to his enemies. 'Let them rot!' he crowed, as appeals were made on behalf of those incarcerated in unspeakable conditions. For the less fortunate, there were still unhappier fates: a show trial and execution, a trip down some stairs in police custody, a homicidal overtaking manoeuvre by an army truck on a quiet road. It is not established that anyone was actually fed to the Shire River crocodiles, but Banda was known to threaten this in moments of poisonous jocosity.

Foreign aid had been plentiful in the Cold War years

when Banda was a steadfast ally against Communism, which he condemned in a short monograph soon after he came to power. But with the collapse of the Soviet Union, this ceased to be important, and the Western democracies tired of his antics. When a group of Catholic bishops was arrested for publishing a denunciation of the regime, Malaŵi's biggest donors pulled the plug.

Things fell apart, and protests were held in the larger cities. Banda's procession, accustomed to being cheered along whole lengths of motorway closed specially for his passage, was pelted in Blantyre as it passed beneath banners celebrating '30 Glorious Years with Kamuzu'.

The regime did not cling stubbornly to power. A radio appeal for order was attempted, though Banda grew confused in the middle of this and missed the key part of the speech. There was an embarrassing altercation on air as an aide cajoled him to try it again, with Banda heard to mumble feebly: 'But I didn't write this.'

The broadcast went unheeded, and Banda soon gave in to calls for a referendum on one-party rule. He was never universally unpopular; to the end, he commanded a substantial core of support, despite losing the referendum and subsequent general election in 1994. A third of the country backed him, but his opponent won with half the votes. Banda conceded defeat even before the results were all in.

Shortly after the referendum, Banda presided over his last Armistice Day service, in honour of the sons of Malaŵi who died for the Allies in the two world wars. November is the peak of the hot season, but a service had been conducted on its eleventh day every year since independence, almost exactly as under the British. Soldiers sweated in scarlet tunics; top brass with ponderous medals sat on a shaded dais; Banda watched rigidly in morning coat, top hat and sunglasses. The military band played 'O God Our Help in Ages Past', and the nonagenarian's lips moved almost imperceptibly as the assembled dignitaries joined in the hymn:

> Thy word commands our flesh to dust,
> 'Return, ye sons of men';
> All nations rose from earth at first,
> And turn to earth again.

The bugle then sounded the Last Post. It might have been a scene from the country's independence ceremony thirty years before, when Prince Philip watched the Union Jack run down and the Malaŵian flag rise in its place. This now hung limply in the windless heat.

The years that followed were unedifying. The new president, Bakili Muluzi, was a man of business who had insinuated himself into Banda's cabinet before launching his own opposition party and usurping his former leader. His ten-year administration is remembered for rapacity shocking even by the standards of the region. During this time, Banda was put on trial for the murder of four MPs killed in a suspicious road 'accident' several years earlier. The case collapsed shortly before his final illness, and he died in hospital in South Africa in 1997. He was almost a hundred years old.

XV

PORTRAIT OF A TYRANT

'Dr Banda built some houses,' my servant Flemings reminisced. 'They were near here, out by the Mzimba road. But people were worried and said, "Dr Banda – these houses are *too* good. They will attract *envy* and *witches* who will make trouble for us." But Dr Banda said: "Don't worry: I have made these houses very strong – so strong that no witches can get inside."' Flemings paused to savour the story's climax. 'And the miracle was that no witches ever got inside.'

Flemings was accompanying me and Dr Highbrow on a return visit to Banda's abandoned palace, Nguru-ya-Nawambe, and we were looking at a scuffed, life-sized oil portrait, propped on the floor against a wall. It showed Banda in sub fusc suit, gold chain of office and the star of the Order of the Lion of Malaŵi. He was standing behind a desk, grasping his chair-back, heavy features on a round, gentle face.

'Normally, a man cannot be one hundred per cent perfect,' Flemings continued, gazing at the painting. 'But the thing about Dr Banda – he *was* one hundred per cent perfect.'

However, the artist had depicted Banda as unexpectedly irresolute before the menacing black clouds which dominated the backdrop of the painting. He looked up and to the side, as if just distracted from his thoughts; eyes, mouth and furrowed brow all bearing a pensive, ambiguous expression.

We were completing our catalogue of the library, and, as often happens, we found that the books furnished their own portrait of the man. We spent three days noting the selections, omissions and a plethora of smaller clues: inscriptions, arrangement, marginalia, dedications, dates and dog-eared pages.

Banda's monogram, present in most of the books, had an interesting evolution to its form. From early on, and for much of his life, he used 'Hastings K. Banda'. Later, amid growing political activity, the European identity was quietened, the African asserted: the style changed to 'H. Kamuzu Banda'.

There was a great quantity of showcase material that might have been bought as a job-lot from an antiquarian bookseller for display purposes only: randomly selected nineteenth-century volumes suggesting no recent use, arranged not by content but by appearance to create a façade of leather-bound erudition. However, such pretension was not the whole; a working part of the collection was separate and cohesive. It did not suggest the unlikely feats of scholarship claimed by his eulogists, but Banda was clearly a serious reader.

Some books, jumbled and neglected, we found in heaps and boxes rather than on the chaotic shelves. Nevertheless, the palimpsest of an original ordering scheme could still be detected. Together in one group were works of history and medicine. The former preponderated and betrayed a preference for the grand narrative over academic detail. The latter were annotated in preparation for exams on surgery and tropical medicine, pharmacology and venereal disease.

However exaggerated the rest of Banda's scholarship may or may not have been, his medical career was serious. In 1937, the president of Eli Lilly, the pharmaceutical company, sent a goodwill present to all doctors graduating from Banda's medical school. It was a copy of the collected wisdom of physician William Osler and was inscribed:

> Dear Doctor:
> Together with congratulations on your attainment of a medical degree, this volume of addresses by Sir William Osler is cordially presented.
> May you catch his vision of the almost boundless possibilities of your chosen profession.
> May you share with him his 'relish of knowledge' and his absorbing love and passionate, persistent search for truth.

There was no doubt self-interest in the giving, but it is startling that even a global corporation should have once been able to express such lofty sentiments. The reference to the 'boundless possibilities' of a career in medicine was ominous: Banda certainly fulfilled that prophecy, though perhaps not in the spirit intended by the dedication. As for the love and search for truth – in this, his achievement was highly ambiguous.

The next part of the collection betrayed Banda's growing interest in politics and the fight against imperialism. Better to understand the mind of the enemy, Banda read studies of colonial administration by authorities of the day. In Lieutenant-Colonel Walter Crocker's *On Governing Colonies*, one passage had been marked:

> The African is improvident to a degree that has no parallel amongst other people. Indeed it is upon his

improvidence that much of his cheerfulness, placidity, idleness, lack of nerves, and physical courage are based. It [. . .] marks all his activities whether as a farmer conserving land or seed, a householder administering the family finances, a lorry driver taking a bend, a domestic lighting a petrol lamp, a soldier engaged in a patrol or advance guard, a journalist writing a political article.

Perhaps this struck a nerve. Banda was punctilious in his affairs and upheld, in his words, 'planning, perfect planning, planning down to the last detail' as the 'secret to success in politics'.

For guidance and inspiration, he seems to have turned to the great figures of history: Peter and Frederick the Great, Mountbatten and Gandhi, Cecil Rhodes and David Livingstone. We also found the memoirs of local friends and enemies – Vorster and Kenyatta, Kaunda and Welensky – felicitously housed as neighbours on the same shelf.

An array of presentation copies contained hand-written dedications, attesting to Malaŵi's eclectic diplomacy: from North Korea, a volume of anti-American propaganda; from Romania, an obscure work of revisionist history by Ceauşescu's little brother; and from the Republic of China, a book of watercolours painted by Madame Chiang Kai-Shek.

Flemings inspected the signature of the Queen of England in a splendidly bound copy of *Royal Heritage*. It did not inspire the same awe as had Banda's, but he was still impressed. Meanwhile, Dr Highbrow noted a fine antique edition of the works of the Roman playwright Terence from the Head Master of Eton College. It was presumably chosen in a spirit of donnish witticism as the author's cognomen was *Afer* – he was 'Terence of Africa'.

There was not much military history, which surprised me. I thought this was essential bedside reading for any dictator, but despite the brutality of his regime, Banda was a mostly peaceable man, not 'greatly interested in armies and fleets', like Auden's tyrant. Nonetheless, his choice of reading during his incarceration by the British in Rhodesia included the campaign diaries of Field Marshal Lord Alanbrooke, bearing the inscription *HKB, HMP Gwelo, 25th December, 1955*. Thus a champion and an enemy of the British Empire were brought strangely together for Christmas in prison, a time about which Banda later jested: 'If the British had really wanted to punish me, they would have had to take away my books.'

It was an earnest collection, but there was a turgor to it, a lack of imagination and levity – with perhaps one exception. The only work of modern fiction was A.J. Cronin's novel *The Citadel*, an account of a young man's struggle to overcome humble origins and become a doctor in Britain in the 1930s. The book was well thumbed, its spine broken, so it fell open on the page describing the protagonist's terror as he contemplates the membership exam for the Royal College of Physicians. In those days, they demanded knowledge of much more than just medicine: 'But the MRCP – it's the most difficult medical exam in the whole shoot. It's – it's *murder*! There's a preliminary paper in four languages. Latin, French, Greek, German. All the Latin I know is dog lingo . . . As for French –'

Cronin's hero passes the exam, thanks to mugging up on Celsus in the original Latin the night before. Banda's own MRCP certificate still hung proudly on the library wall. I thought of his pronouncement: 'To me, to call a man B.A., M.A., when he does not know a single word of Latin, is deceiving people.' A few years after he said this, Kamuzu

Academy and then the Classics department at the University of Malaŵi opened for business.

Banda certainly studied Latin in America, but it is not clear that he learnt very much, nor any Greek. Only translations in either language bore signs of use. An absence of dictionaries, grammars, primers and lexicons argued against the collection of a linguist.

But it did look as if Banda returned to Classics in later life. From the 1970s onwards, there were more and more editions of the Greek and Roman authors, albeit mostly in English. The condition of spines and pages suggested spasmodic forays rather than assiduous study. Reading of the poets and philosophers, in particular, looked to have been abandoned quickly. But the historians had been tackled determinedly. There were a dozen copies of *The Gallic Wars* alone – including the 1584 Manutius Press edition. Why so much Caesar? It suggested some powerful and important symbolism operating on the collector's mind.

XVI

THE DIALECT OF THE TRIBE

At the opening of Kamuzu Academy in 1981, Banda addressed an immense crowd of pupils and masters, villagers and assembled dignitaries. After a lengthy exposition of his peasant upbringing and the importance of classical education, he then proceeded to declaim page after page of Caesar's *Gallic Wars* – in the original Latin – beginning '*Gallia est omnis divisa in partes tres . . .*'

Until this point he had spoken in English, with an aide translating into Chichewa. When the flow of Latin finally ceased, the crowd was told simply: '*Mwamva zimene amene Kamuzu!*' – 'You heard what Kamuzu said!'

Boaters and blazers stood proud in the sun. An honour guard snapped to attention. Ngoni warriors gestured their obeisance with ox-hide shields and spears. Masked *gule* dancers cavorted wildly amid the roar of the crowd and the paeans of the dancing women.

Such exhibitionism invites uncomfortable parallels. A few years earlier, two of Banda's peers were overthrown: Idi Amin and Jean-Bédel Bokassa. As President of Uganda, Amin was famous for mimicking the Scottish officers who had kicked him about while he was still a regimental cookboy. Fancying himself 'The Last King of Scotland', he sported a kilt and as many medals as could be pinned to his gargantuan chest. So attired, he took the salute from massed regiments attired as Highlanders, marching past to the sound of bagpipes, fifes and drums.

Meanwhile Bokassa redesignated the Central African Republic as an 'Empire', crowning himself and his consort in a ceremony modelled on Napoleon's coronation, complete with an escort of cavalry in plumed shakos and gold braid last seen at Waterloo. He could have stepped out of the portrait by Ingres: ermine-clad, bejewelled, with sceptre and diadem, seated on a vast imperial throne. The spectacle cost more than the country's entire incoming aid budget. Within a few years, both Uganda and the Central African Empire had disintegrated in welters of genocide, war and – it was widely reported – cannibalism.

It has been well argued – most famously by Frantz Fanon – that the real damage of colonialism was psychological. It fostered inferiority complexes and megalomania that blighted the continent's post-independence leadership. There is a trace of this in Banda, especially when he chose to belabour his audience in Latin, which nobody present could understand. The episode recalls another painful occasion, soon after his return home, when one of his countrymen approached Banda with bare feet: 'Get that disgusting man out of my sight!' is said to have been his horrified response.

Nevertheless, Banda's mentality was not the same as Amin's or Bokassa's. Despite glimpses of their mimicry, Banda was intelligent, educated, worldly. Sure, Classics had its symbolic, even fetishistic importance for him, as it did for me, but it also meant much more: the subject granted access to a culture which might otherwise have eluded us. And unlike Amin and Bokassa, Banda wanted others to benefit from what he had enjoyed. Education would instil Malawians with the confidence to engage with the wider world. In Western high culture, Banda saw a path to equality.

The striking counterpoint to this was that Banda was also vigorous in promoting the indigenous culture of Malaŵi. Early on, he made a prominent show of support at the installation of Paramount Chief Lundu, treating the crowd to a lengthy historical discourse on the tribes of Malaŵi, their origins, migrations and kings. This gesture was the start of a sustained programme of patronage of traditional rulers. Chiefs at every level were accorded public respect by Banda, and thereby dignified in the eyes of their people. Executive and judicial powers were devolved to 'Traditional Authorities', village courts and local headmen, who communicated Banda's supreme sanction of village custom. Above all, farmers were to be cherished as the bedrock of the country's identity. Malaŵi had no natural resources except the soil, and Banda was fond of suggesting this might be no bad thing.

Regulation of language became central to Banda's cultural vision. When he was in England, he met a visiting chief from his home district and was dismayed to find he struggled to communicate with him in their shared mother tongue. But Banda reached a characteristically defiant conclusion. It was not that his command of Chichewa had dwindled during his forty years abroad. On the contrary, when he left home he had carried with him a pure version of the language, which had become corrupted in his absence. British colonialists were sloppy in their usage, and complaisant Malaŵians had first tolerated, then assimilated, their errors. The result was a debased pidgin. Living abroad, Banda had been insulated from this degeneracy, leaving him the sole custodian of true Chichewa.

A committee was set up 'to purify the dialect of the tribe'. Grammar and orthography were standardised, and any points of uncertainty or inconsistency settled by presidential fiat. Proper pronunciation was safeguarded by a new system of accentuation. The name Malaŵi was not to be pronounced with a mere 'w' or 'v'. The consonant now represented by 'ŵ' denoted a voiced bilabial fricative, he took pains to emphasise. At the opening of the country's first university, he addressed the newly appointed academics as their chancellor. Splendidly attired in black and gold bonnet, hood and gown, he berated them on the parlous misuse of language by their countrymen: 'Don't be having an inferiority complex about this – correct the white man if he gets things wrong!'

Their duty was to arrest the process of degradation, but, to do this properly, they would need Latin as a framework for thinking critically about their own language. To start them in their task, he gave a lengthy address on Chichewa grammar, which he delivered in English, with supporting examples from Latin. The corresponding Chichewa examples were drawn from specially chosen fragments of traditional song performed by his dancing women. Thus, when Banda compared the subjunctive in Bantu languages with that in Latin, he would signal to the women to illustrate his point. The audience blinked in bafflement, and a diffident minister offered a low-brow translation for the humbler listeners, based on what he had taken from the songs: 'His Excellency is now talking about groundnuts.'

There is much that is perverse in this, but also something important and sincere. Forty years of separation had made Banda desperate to recover the culture he had lost. And forty years in the West had persuaded him how easily that culture might be corroded once the outside world began to intrude.

'More paternalistic than the British' was an accusation sometimes levelled at Banda. And indeed he felt that his countrymen were too innocent of modernity to judge for themselves the good and evil thereof. Television was obviously a pernicious influence, and so Malaŵi was spared its introduction until 1996. Other media were also heavily censored. An extensive catalogue of prohibited material identified a wide array of corrupting influences: John Berger, the *Emmanuelle* film series, Simone de Beauvoir, Orwell, Nabokov and the music of Paul Simon. Numerous decadent aliens were variously persecuted, with Jehovah's Witnesses particularly singled out, and even occasionally murdered by overenthusiastic *gule wamkulu* dancers. At one time or another, Banda also expelled hippies, liberal journalists, the US Peace Corps, women with exposed knees and men with hair below the collar line. 'If that is Western Civilisation, you can keep it in America,' he muttered disgustedly.

Indecorous tourists were eyed suspiciously on arrival by zealous immigration officials and either turned back, compelled to dress properly, or subjected to an involuntary short-back-and-sides. In a spasm of revulsion, Banda decreed that bell-bottom trousers should never see the light of day in Malaŵi. A team of legislators began furiously working through the details of the new law. One later admitted it had proved a challenging task, involving long and careful comparison of his colleagues' wardrobes. Eventually they devised a formulation that met all moral, legal and practical desiderata: 'For the purposes of the Act, the expression "bell-bottom trousers" means any flared trousers so made that the circumference of each leg thereof measured along the bottom edge is greater than six fifths of the circumference of such leg measured at its narrowest point parallel to the aforesaid bottom edge.'

It is easy to mock, but the context is important. In 1976, as political conditions in nearby countries reached a crescendo of cruelty, mayhem, injustice and slaughter,

Banda's Malaŵi Congress Party was ratifying a *relatively* gentle programme of quixotic conservatism. Power was devolved to the villages. They were to encourage discussion of morals and standards of behaviour. Decency in dress and deportment were celebrated. The old tribal initiation rites were to be preserved. For the men of his own Chewa people, this meant initiation into Nyau – the dancers of *gule wamkulu*.

The great mystery is whether or not Banda was himself initiated as a teenager before he left home. Villagers from his home district, like Sangala, told me that it would in those days have been impossible for a young boy to avoid it. And in the introduction which Banda wrote to a book on Malaŵian custom, he states that you cannot be fully a man if you have not been initiated. On the other hand, Banda never spoke of this, not even to his companion of thirty years, Mama Kadzamira. You sense a tension, as though European and African identities were so delicately balanced that the question of his initiation would, if answered, tilt him irrevocably into one camp or the other.

Banda made use of his ambiguous status to set himself above his compatriots. 'I am not just another African. I am Kamuzu,' he pronounced haughtily. This detachment allowed him to steer Malaŵi away from the sort of tribalism that so often vitiated politics elsewhere, but it issued from deep, personal isolation.

On his return to Malaŵi, distant relatives were sought out and accorded respect, but it is not clear that real intimacy was established. After leaving Europe, Banda seems to have made few – if any – close friends. In London, he had had a long affair with a married woman, but when Merene French divorced her husband in expectation of a life with Banda, he hesitated. The agony of Seretse Khama, first President of Botswana, and his English wife Ruth Williams was still very current: their marriage had scandalised people in both Britain and Botswana. As an aspiring black nationalist politician, Banda feared provoking the same reaction. Details are scant, but the affair seems to have ended painfully.

His sense of alienation rings clear from a tortured letter he wrote while living in Britain but thinking of home. 'No Nyasaland girl could be a real companion for me,' he confessed. 'Of course, I am a Chewa. But my long sojourn [abroad] has so completely changed my outlook on life, that any girl in Nyasaland is, in reality, a foreigner to me.' He did eventually form a lasting friendship with Kadzamira, but it remains uncertain whether it ever amounted to more than that.

'This profoundly lonely man, locked in the prison-house of power,' was the judgement of the Church of Scotland when its elders wrote in criticism of his government in the 1990s. And indeed 'I'm so lonely' is rumoured to have been Banda's near final utterance. In a land where the bonds of kith and kin seem everywhere so obvious, natural and strong, Banda's isolation appears even more stark. He obsessed about belonging because he knew that he did not. 'Learn English, learn Latin, yes! But first learn your own village ways,' he warned. 'Without these, you will be lost, quite lost.'

XVII

DE RADICULIS

Kamuzu means 'Little Roots', appropriately enough. Banda's mother chose the name in honour of a herbalist whose remedy had cured her of infertility and given her a son. But when Banda returned to Malaŵi after forty years abroad, the land of his birth was an unfamiliar place. Even among the country's educated few, he stood out with his unusual experience and sophistication. To the great mass of rural poor, he might have come from the moon. He looked different, sounded different, barely spoke the same language. In dress and deportment, he was British, urbane, even patrician. He favoured European food, ate with cutlery, read books. His manners were genteel, and he liked to use a proper bathroom. The latter seems to have been a particular source of anxiety during political campaigns, when he conducted long tours of remote provinces. In the early days – before a string of comfortable residences had been acquired – Banda's agents would be sent ahead to reconnoitre sanitary arrangements up-country.

Yet despite the cultural dissonance, this was the reunion he had yearned for. Back in his 'home district', Banda went in search of his roots. He was desperate to find the graves of his parents, both of whom had died during his long absence abroad, but he could locate neither. Distant relatives remembered too little. Who even were his parents?

His mother's identity was fairly well established, but his father's was more mysterious. Was he even of the same tribe as her?

From the palace on the hill, you ought to be able to make out the village where Banda was born, somewhere among the numberless mud-brick dwellings scattered over the landscape. But there is some dispute about its location. When I asked Flemings, Sangala and various local headmen, they all gave very firm, very inconsistent answers. The time of Banda's birth was also unsettled: it was in the late 1890s, but he could not be sure of the year, let alone the day.

As if to make up for all this uncertainty, Banda made much of the places that he *could* identify: villages that he remembered, wells where he had drunk, remarkable trees – all were formally memorialized. Kamuzu Academy was of course founded specifically on the site of his boyhood school. And then there was the hill where he built his palace.

Banda had been carried there as a child on his grandfather's shoulders. The old man had wanted to point out the slope where, in his own lifetime, a great battle had been fought against the Ngoni, a warrior tribe who had broken away from Shaka's Zulus and marauded north, devastating the region. The site of the battle became known as Nguru-ya-Nawambe: 'the place where Nawambe lost his shield'. Nawambe was a corruption of Ndabambi – the name of the Ngoni chief whom Banda's peaceable Chewa tribe had unexpectedly defeated. But for that victory, his ancestors might all have been wiped out.

It was the natural location for the palace: the scene of his people's courage, sacrifice and unlikely deliverance from destruction. And it was also a childhood memory, a tradition transmitted orally by his elders, something of his own heritage that he could personally lay claim to. But today the battle of Nguru-ya-Nawambe is fading from popular consciousness. I tried asking about it in the local area but encountered mostly blankness. I had to seek out the aged Ngoni historian, D.D. Phiri, for the etymology of the name. This was presumably what Banda had feared: history slipping from your grasp. The palace was intended to serve as a memorial. As such, *The Gallic Wars* was its perfect adornment.

Habent sua fata libelli: books have their own destinies. So jested a late Roman grammarian, noting the fickleness by which some works are lost, others preserved for posterity. The saying evoked the Dark Ages in Europe but seemed even more resonant at Nguru-ya-Nawambe. A few hundred years after Caesar, the Roman Empire fell and literature almost disappeared from Europe. Over the following centuries, only a few manuscripts survived in those rare corners where civilisation sheltered. In the Renaissance, the texts were rescued by the great pioneers of printing, whereupon *The Gallic Wars* became one of the most widely read books in the world. It was a manual for princes and generals, but also for Classics students, because of its simple, soldierly style. Until recently it was usually the first work of original Latin introduced to school pupils, its ubiquity such that even Asterix could allude to it in jokes. However, by the time I studied Classics, *The Gallic Wars* had fallen out of favour. We translated excerpts, but none of us read well enough to get through the whole thing. After two millennia of survival by the skin of its teeth, it seemed as if the book might be consigned to obscurity by the information age.

In Malaŵi, however, Banda insisted on its value even as Europe neglected it. He presumably took a dictator's pride in identifying himself with Caesar. Returning to Africa to lead his people must have felt like his own crossing of the Rubicon, his defiance of the colonial state like the battle for supremacy in Republican Rome. But I suspect his interest was also subtler than that.

Caesar's *Gallic Wars* relate the author's campaigns against the tribes of modern-day France, Germany and Britain in the first century BC. There is much on the people and their customs, observed with the imperialist's eye but still curious and even sympathetic. Crucially, it describes a period when Western Europe was a land of barbarians awaiting foreign civilisation. Banda wanted Africans to know about this, and Europeans never to forget it.

'You were under Roman management then!' he reminded the outgoing colonial administrators in an impromptu history lesson just after he assumed power. *The Gallic Wars* was more than just a symbol of the Western culture Banda admired and had assimilated. It also related facts that subverted the authority of his country's oppressors.

Above all, though, Caesar stood for the miracle of *written* history. So much of Banda's own heritage had been lost and forgotten in only a few decades, while *The Gallic Wars* still preserved the record of distant millennia. I contemplated the volume again. As an object, it was highly desirable: exquisite in design and manufacture, and in near perfect condition. I felt an almost overwhelming temptation to 'rescue' it from the abandoned palace. But it seemed to whisper that Nguru-ya-Nawambe was its rightful resting place, that it was a talisman, there to protect the hill and its story from the forces of oblivion. I put the book back in its chest and returned it to the library. However, seeking a romantic gesture, I did permit myself one small act of theft: I took an old cigarette from the silver box on the desk, presumably intended for guests. I lit it and gazed out over the battlefield. The tobacco was stale and rather disgusting, but, as the smoke rose upwards in the still air, I imagined the Shade of Caesar presiding over the place.

PART THREE
ONLY CONNECT

XVIII

IN WESTMINSTER ABBEY

When Banda first visited London, he went straight to Westminster Abbey, where he startled onlookers by speaking out loud to the tomb of David Livingstone: 'Dr Livingstone, it is I, Kamuzu Banda from Kasungu, Nyasaland. I will go back to Nyasaland one day to take up your work; I promise.' With his customary alertness to history, Banda was echoing Livingstone's famous words when he addressed the students of Oxford and Cambridge in 1857. It was the speech in which he implored the undergraduates to go to Central Africa and join his campaign to establish Christianity, Commerce and Civilisation in place of slavery.

These values trouble us now, but, for Banda and many Malaŵians, Livingstone and his achievements were unequivocally good things. Moreover, the men who followed Livingstone were the first to create the atmosphere of intellectual curiosity that has suffused Malaŵi's history ever since. My own interest is stirred by their attempts to reach out towards the alien culture they encountered. Their story is now largely forgotten, but we in the West would do well to re-examine it. In our pursuit of multicultural ideals, we today stand in their shadow.

Livingstone spent the years 1851 to 1873 exploring Central Africa, travelling mostly on foot in areas previously visited by few, if any, Europeans. In the territory of modern Malaŵi, he found a land of great fertility whose societies were in turmoil. Long before Livingstone, a pygmy people once dwelt in the region, but they were slowly supplanted and exterminated by waves of Bantu migrants from the Congo basin. Whenever I drove to the capital, I passed the lonely mountain where the last of the pygmies were said to have been flushed out of their hiding places and killed.

The newcomers dwelt in conditions of apparent prosperity beside Lake Malaŵi for a number of centuries. Yet by the time of Livingstone's arrival, their existence was threatened. The Ngoni had migrated from southern Africa and were scattering, enslaving, raping or murdering everyone they met along the way. Settled agricultural practices were disrupted by the chaos, leading to perennial famine. It was described as a land of starving, mutilated people eking out a living amid torched villages and rivers choked with corpses.

Malaŵi was also at the heart of the Indian Ocean slave trade, in which the Arabs, the Portuguese and local African tribes had been engaged for many centuries. The peoples of Lake Malaŵi were the principal pool from which slaves were drawn, the business model already well established when Livingstone encountered it. Tribes who had converted to Islam, especially the Yao, did most of the hard work: they raided the villages of other tribes, yoking and manacling anyone it was not more expedient to put to death. Then they forced them to march to the coast, a journey of at least 400 miles. With logs fixed around their necks, malnourished and abused, and bearing impossible loads over difficult and dangerous terrain, many perished in transit. But the supply must have been so plentiful, and the demand so great, as to make this loss financially acceptable. Once at the coast, middle men bought the survivors at a cost of, for example, four yards of calico for a ten-year-old boy. They then conveyed their purchases to slave markets, the largest of which was for a long time at Zanzibar. From here the slaves were sold on to buyers from the Middle East, the Swahili Coast, the plantation islands of the Indian Ocean, and beyond.

There have been fashionable glosses on this trade over the last fifty years, especially insisting that it was less pernicious than its transatlantic equivalent. But even allowing for every well-reasoned revision, the situation which Livingstone described in the territory of Malaŵi in the 1850s and 1860s sounds like hell on earth. It always used to perplex me how a handful of missionaries could, without force, have converted such a great swathe of the world to a new religion. The answer lies partly in the conditions of horror that had long prevailed there. When outsiders appeared proposing peace on earth and goodwill to all men, their message was embraced enthusiastically.

The infamous 'Three Cs' embarrass us today. Christianity drifts further from relevance, while the merits of commerce seem more and more doubtful. As for Western civilisation, its mere mention can call to mind Gandhi's *bon mot*: that 'it would be a good idea'. The taint of colonialism is highly toxic, and Livingstone and his project have fallen far from grace. They may yet fall further, if recent events in Britain and America are anything to go by. But before we pass ever harsher judgements on the past, we must try to educate ourselves: the context is essential.

Several years after I left Malaŵi, I visited Blantyre in Scotland (after which Malaŵi's commercial capital is named). It is the site of the nineteenth-century cotton mill where Livingstone grew up. I took a train south-east from Glasgow and then made my way along terraces of pebble-dash and PVC windows, past a pub doing a brisk late-morning trade and a newsagent, outside which young mothers rocked prams and shared Superkings. On a small billboard, the headline of a local paper alluded to the recent scandal of a woman kicked in the stomach by the father of her unborn child in a rage fuelled by Buckfast.

Eventually I arrived at the gates of the whitewashed tenement where the Livingstone family had once made their home. Theirs had been a single room on the second floor in which parents and seven children cohabited, cooking, sleeping and drawing water every day on yokes up a steep spiral staircase. The family had moved there from the Hebridean island of Ulva, where they had lived in conditions that must have made Blantyre seem an earthly paradise. Whereas before they had struggled to subsist off an icy, barren, windswept smallholding, now there was at least paid employment and lodging for all. Aged ten, Livingstone began twelve-hour working days, employed to dart among the moving parts of the spinning jenny to tie up the broken threads of cotton.

It was a large profit-making concern, but the mill owner had a high-minded conception of the possibilities of improvement for his staff. Beside the factories were a school, hospital and library, which he sponsored. Livingstone began borrowing books, and, when he became a spinner, learned to balance these precariously on the monstrous machine he was operating. When he returned to his parents' room each night, he embarked on further homework, and was thereby able to teach himself the fundamentals of Latin, Greek, theology and the sciences. On display in his room are the copies of Horace and Vergil that he read in the original Latin – texts which students struggle with today, even after four years at university.

As is well known, Livingstone trained as a medical missionary, was sent to Africa, explored its most uncharted recesses, and campaigned tirelessly for its improvement. His plan was to eliminate slavery and, in its place, recreate the same austere but uplifting conditions by which he (and all his siblings) had improved themselves in Scotland. If that vision makes us uncomfortable, it may be because our own age has made a tragic mockery of the idea that work will set you free. Raised as he was, Livingstone had no such misgivings. As he hacked his way through trails in Central Africa, he was fond of singing Robert Burns' 'Is There for Honest Poverty':

> Then let us pray that come it may,
>   (As come it will for a' that,)
>
> [. . .] That Man to Man, the world o'er,
>   Shall brothers be for a' that!

Livingstone's memory is cherished today throughout the region he explored. Anniversaries are celebrated, the trees beneath which he preached are venerated as national monuments, and his hometown in Scotland is the object of pilgrimage. D.D. Phiri wrote movingly of his own visit there. Would his people even exist, he was prompted to ask, were it not for Livingstone? As a schoolboy, Phiri remembered getting his lessons mixed up: the Holy Land was surely Scotland, and the humble Glasgow suburb of Blantyre became Nazareth.

XIX

VITAÏ LAMPADA

In the event, Livingstone enacted very little of his vision. He was a lonely pioneer, more mystic or fanatic than builder, but when he returned to Britain he was determined to recruit others to his cause. On the seas, the Royal Navy had been suppressing slavery by force since 1815. Now Livingstone wanted missionaries to target the source of the trade – the area centred around Malaŵi that he referred to as the 'open sore' of the world. 'I beg to direct your attention to Africa', he appealed to the Cambridge Union. 'Carry out the work which I have begun!' The students cheered him, took up his challenge and, in so doing, committed themselves to self-immolation.

Volunteers from Oxbridge, Durham and Trinity College Dublin formed the UMCA – the Universities' Mission to Central Africa. Other missions were also founded (especially from Scotland), to which hundreds of young men and women signed up. They sailed to the coast of East Africa and then began the long, difficult journey on foot to the interior. They knew they were approaching their destination as the traffic of passing slave caravans became denser. Arrival was marked by the omnipresence of shattered villages and terrorised people.

Two hundred volunteered for the Universities' Mission alone, of whom fifty-seven died in this service – a higher mortality rate than at the Somme. Malaria and dysentery claimed the most victims, but the missionaries also had to contend with countless other tropical diseases, accidents and misadventure, man-slaying beasts of the forest, the enmity of slavers and the suspicion of warlike tribes. A few seem also to have succumbed to loneliness and despair.

Different tactics were employed over a thirty-year period. An early attempt at armed confrontation with the slavers ended in disaster, with the mission's militant first bishop, Charles Mackenzie, left buried in a hastily dug grave at the mouth of the Ruo River. Thereafter, the main approach was the foundation of remote stations, where rescued and runaway slaves could be sheltered. Success was achieved mostly through a heroic appeal to better nature, bolstered by demonstration of the fruits of modern medicine and education, for which an immense appetite soon emerged. Beyond the mission stations, other missionaries undertook solitary work, wandering among the local peoples, and attempting gentle persuasion on any who would listen.

By 1896, the last slaver fiefdoms had been extirpated from the territory of present-day Malaŵi. One was defeated only after a nightmarish seven-year war of attrition, fought by just a few dozen men in a beleaguered stockade on the northern lakeshore, but this was unusual. Slavery in the interior was ended for the most part peaceably and with only limited help from the British government.

I am a member of no church, and this is not a work of or about the propagation of Christianity. But the elimination of slavery from Central Africa by these young men strikes me as among the greatest moral achievements of modern times. I can think of no other that was made without compulsion, to so great effect, and in a spirit of such self-sacrifice.

Chauncy Maples and William Johnson were friends at Oxford. In his final year at the university, Johnson emerged from a Sanskrit tutorial to find an appeal for missionaries to Central Africa pinned on the college noticeboard. He already had an offer of work with the Indian Civil Service, the nineteenth-century equivalent of a place on J.P. Morgan's fast-track graduate programme. ('The heaven-born' was how these men were known in British India.) As Maples observed, his friend could look forward to 'a thousand a year, infinite chances of promotion, altogether one of the finest openings (from a worldly point of view) that a young man can have'.

Educated at Bedford Grammar School, Johnson was of middle-class origins, and might have been expected to want to better himself socially and financially. But he turned the job down and signed up instead for mission work. His courage stirred Maples to do the same, and the two immediately set about the important work of choosing epitaphs, in expectation that they might shortly find their graves in Africa.

On the long voyage from England, both went down with fever even before touching the continent's mainland. They spent a year in Zanzibar, adjusting to conditions, during which both became seriously ill. Indeed, Johnson was told to go home: his doctor concluded that his constitution was too weak for Africa, and that he could not hope to survive there. Undiscouraged, they gathered their strength before embarking on the journey from the coast. Their initial goal was the mission station at Masasi, 400 miles away in modern-day Tanzania. On the way, Johnson began to develop the chronic tropical sores on his arms and legs which would afflict him his whole life in Africa.

From Masasi, he set off in the direction of Lake Malawî with a small train of porters. He was then joined by another friend, Charles Janson, who had just arrived from Oxford. Janson fell ill almost immediately, but they jollied along nevertheless, delightedly quoting Xenophon when at last they caught sight of the lake. But one day their shelter was flooded in torrential rains, and they lost the greater part of their stores. Then it became clear that Janson was getting much worse.

They were trying to hack their way back to the mission, but it was the rainy season, so rivers were high. Their retreat got slower and slower until, many miles from help, Janson became too ill to continue: Johnson's impression was that he had contracted cholera. Forced to stop for rest, they at first raised their spirits by attempting to reconstruct the original Greek of Saint Paul's *Epistle to the Romans*. But Janson's diarrhoea and vomiting became profuse, and his friend had to devote all his energies to nursing him. The only remedies they had left were brandy and laudanum, which, they noticed, seemed to make the symptoms worse. After a few days, Janson died, having lasted only three weeks in Africa. Johnson dug a grave in some loose sand and resumed his mission. He wrote in his journal: 'Charles Janson left us on Shrove Tuesday 1882, and I went on up the coast alone in that Lenten season [. . .] We are for the time parted, but I don't think God leaves gaps long in such work as this.'

He was in fact proved very wrong: Johnson survived another forty-six years in Africa, most of them spent wandering around Lake Malaŵi, which, it is worth remembering, is 360 miles long. At first he travelled alone, evangelising where he was welcomed, mocked and pelted with maize cobs where he was not. Then he contracted a destructive tropical eye infection and went almost completely blind, whereafter a servant had to guide him on his travels. He made a lonely base at Liuli on the lake's northeastern shore, in modern-day Tanzania. There he built a small church and kept a grass hut for himself, but he was mostly itinerant, travelling with just a bundle of clothes, a reed mat, an earthenware pot, his pens and his books. He lived as a mendicant, which, in a land racked by famine, frequently meant just a meal of beans a day if he was lucky.

Of course there was *Boys' Own* adventure to his travels: he was attacked by a lion and imprisoned by the slaver Chief Makanjila. The former relented, and the latter released him unharmed, apparently because his saintly forbearance suggested so little a threat. One of his jailers became a convert and, in later life, would participate in Edward VII's coronation in London as a soldier of the King's African Rifles.

More striking than the derring-do is the solitude and determination of Johnson's engagement with the world around him. He mapped the terrain and recorded its flora. He acquired local lore and the skills to survive. Above all, he studied the indigenous languages. He had been a linguist at Oxford, acquiring Latin, Greek, Hebrew, Sanskrit, French and Arabic. When he met imams on his travels, he would jump excitedly at the chance to discuss the Koran, which he always carried with him. But more often than not he was disappointed, and grumbled like an Oxford don about their poor command of Arabic. It was with local languages that his achievement most astonishes: he mastered at least six, and translated the Bible and Book of Common Prayer into Chinyanja.

There is a totality to Johnson's immersion in the local culture that you would think possible only by complete effacement of his original self. Yet his core was changeless. No doubt he owed most to his Christian faith; but you also detect, here and there in his writing, the odd reference to another culture he knew. In a lyrical passage in his

Reminiscences, scenes from Africa stir still earlier memories as he writes of 'Homeric aspects of the lake'. In his mind's eye, Likoma evokes the isles of Greece; Mang'anja canoes, painted red and black, become the ships of Odysseus; a Yao chief's funeral that of Patroclus in the *Iliad*; an Ngoni warrior with spear and panther's skin is Achilles; and a limping, hapless archer the sorrowful Philoctetes.

But the proof of Johnson's engagement was in the love shown him by the peoples of the lakeshore. It was not long before he could wander fearlessly among usually implacable tribes, and he even came to be celebrated in local song. One hailed him as 'the Socrates of the lake', presumably from what he had taught his parishioners of the classical world. His memory is still cherished, and the people of his former parish continue to celebrate 'Saint Johnson's Day', despite official contestation of his sainthood by Lambeth Palace. At Liuli, where he died aged eighty-nine – still hard at work – his grave remains venerated.

'Wherever sympathetic study is given,' Johnson observed of his language work, 'you will find affinities in all directions.'

'Look fixedly on man, as man, anywhere, and long vistas of ideas will open before you.'

XX

EVEN UNTO DEATH

Johnson's friend Maples gave his life much earlier. After his first mission station was overrun by an Ngoni war party, a decision was made to relocate to the island of Likoma on Lake Malaŵi, where a small community could be kindled to life in safety. This was his great work: at the spot on the island where he had come across three witches being burned alive, Maples built a church. No witch was ever burned there again, and the community flourished.

Johnson and Maples were very different: the former lived a life of wandering, solitude, contemplation; the latter was a builder, administrator and leader of men. They remained best friends, and Johnson would periodically retreat to Likoma on breaks from his meanderings, rejoicing briefly in rest, safety, companionship and Hebrew word games. Maples was somewhat mercurial: he was a practical man, who enjoyed constructing artesian wells and fashioning his own dug-out canoes; but he also delighted in cookery and conjuring, as well as in Chaucer, Milton and Wordsworth. He composed the only sonnet dedicated to Lake Malaŵi, just before it claimed his life. Its words proved hauntingly prophetic:

> [. . .] Cerulean Lake! Let this thy mission be
> To speak to us of Him, who in His hand
> Thy waters broad uplifts; and so may we,
> While lingering on our pilgrimage, a land,
> Not bounded by earth's limits, ever see
> But far above her mists – the Heavenly strand.

Maples was consecrated Bishop of Likoma in 1895 but, during his short absence, a close colleague died of blackwater fever, and another was speared to death. Learning of this on his return journey, Maples hurriedly set sail from the western lakeshore to restore order in the diocese, but his boat capsized in a storm and he was drowned.

This episode was uncomfortably on my mind as I made my own crossing to Likoma. The only boat going that day was little more than an oversized dinghy, made of flimsy timbers, unshielded from the sun and resembling the worst sort of vessel in news footage of the Mediterranean migrant crisis. There was a single outboard motor of a size intended only to power a small rib, and a crowd of about twenty passengers waiting to embark, all associated with a mountain of cargo piled messily on the beach: car tyres, engine parts, sacks of rice and potatoes, medical supplies, timber and cement. I was there before six, but two hours passed in indecision about whether the boat would leave at all. When embarkation finally began, this took up the rest of the morning as everyone scrabbled and argued about their space on board. The process was interrupted by a rumour that the crew did not have enough diesel for the journey. Loading was suspended, and an hour given over to bickering and recrimination. At length a decrepit 4x4 crawled down to the lakeshore, and a couple of jerry cans of fuel were surrendered.

As the boat was loaded, it began to slant more and more heavily towards the starboard side, until this sat just a foot above the surface of the water. Passengers were crammed wherever space allowed, mostly on top of the cargo, which had been randomly arranged and covered with a rough tarpaulin. I counted myself lucky to have found a perch on a slender beam of wood, wedged between two other passengers with my feet dangling carefully to avoid stepping on a woman lying below on bags of bruised vegetables.

Just before noon, the motor was at last tried, but failed to start. The sun was beating down hard; I put a scarf over my head and sweated it out. The engine was dismantled, important-looking parts were removed and balanced precariously on the side of the bobbing vessel. The engine was reassembled, retested, disassembled, reassembled. I became sure the boat was fundamentally unseaworthy and resolved to abandon my trip if the problem was not fixed in half an hour. I was gazing at my watch when, with five minutes to spare, the engine jumped to life. I had an immediate sickening feeling in the pit of my stomach.

Weren't we too late to be starting? Likoma was forty miles across the lake. But everyone reassured themselves: it was, by the skipper's estimate, only a four- to five-hour crossing. We should be there around nightfall.

We chugged slowly out of the harbour with an unhappy-sounding engine propelling us at about a walking pace. In open water, it became clear that the wind was against us, and that this would be our top speed. Estimates for the journey time were revised to between six and seven hours. Before the last bar of mobile signal disappeared, I made a rough calculation based on my phone's fading GPS tracker and realised this was out of the question.

The next ten hours were not happy. Hot and cramped, I rationed my drinking water. After four hours, we were still in sight of the shore we had left while Likoma remained out of sight. An hour later there was muted jubilation as the island was identified as a minute speck on the far horizon. And then the sun set, plunging us into total darkness.

It grew cold, the wind picked up, and the lake became rough. The pilot had earlier been able to direct the boat so it took the waves head on with minimal rolling. With visibility now nil and the water much choppier, this became impossible. At one point a crew member tried leaning from the prow with his phone torch to illuminate the course of the waves but quickly gave up. We began to bob more and more violently; one passenger repositioned himself so he could vomit overboard for the rest of the journey.

We had hit a storm. Every few minutes a wave would strike us hard, water would splash into the side of the boat, and the passengers would scream. I looked around to identify some item of buoyant cargo that I might grab hold of if we went down, and I took note of the position of the stars so I might not paddle in completely the wrong direction if I found myself in the water. But I was not sanguine: we were twenty miles from either shore, and it would be days before anyone noticed our boat was missing. And who could or would look for us when they did?

I thought of Maples attempting the same crossing and wondered at his strength of character. I spent most of that journey resentful of my discomfort and fearful for my safety. But Maples, the young man who claimed to be a coward, died a hero. When the waters capsized his boat, and the passengers were thrashing about in the storm-tossed water, he realised his episcopal cassock was weighing down the flotsam to which they were all clinging. And so he detached himself from the party, bidding them to save themselves, and sank beneath the waves.

We arrived on Likoma around midnight, and I felt silly for having been so scared.

The next day revealed a tropical paradise set in windless calm beneath a perfect blue sky. Likoma is set in crystal-clear waters, with silver sand beaches nestled in green bays. Its small town rings with Caribbean cheer, and the people rejoice in the relative wealth generated by the country's best supply of fish. Just behind the town lies Saint Peter's Cathedral – one of the finest churches I have seen anywhere.

It has not the crushing immensity of a European cathedral, but its crenellated walls and tower are still hefty, evoking its history as a refuge from slavers and warrior tribes on the mainland. Likoma's architects were inspired by Iona, the island abbey in the Hebrides, founded as a corner of safety against the turmoil of the Dark Ages. Both possess an atmosphere of sanctuary, with stern exteriors sheltering serene inner cloisters. But unlike its Scottish antecedent, Saint Peter's is adorned with palm trees and beds of dense mauve flowers, basking in the light which glows from the soft yellow stone of baptistery, belfry and library.

Most of the building work was completed after Maples' death, but Johnson lived to see it finished, albeit only through his one less afflicted eye, darkly. Yet both men are evoked by the place: in its strangeness and gentleness, its atmosphere of learning and meditation, and in its bewildering union of styles.

Tropical sun showered through stained glass to produce a psychedelic version of High Gothic, all bathed in the refulgent sound of an African women's choir, who were rehearsing during my visit. They sang a psalm of exuberant melody, drummed to a fast processional rhythm, as I wandered among the cathedral's treasures. An episcopal throne might have been lifted from Westminster Abbey, diaconal pews from the Garter Chapel at Windsor, but soapstone carvings all around somehow suggested the African and Celtic simultaneously, while the baptismal font, built for total immersion, would have felt at home in a church of militant Romanesque. Even the Orthodox was represented: there were images of saints in the style of Greek icons, while an Ethiopian crozier was displayed opposite that of Mackenzie, first bishop of the Universities' Mission, who died downriver from the lake. There was a movingly carved black Madonna, Ngoni ivory, a stone from Canterbury, sculptures from Oberammergau, bells from Ludgate. Perhaps the proudest relic was a crucifix of wood from the tree at Ilala in Zambia, beneath which Livingstone's heart is buried. A chapel was studded with memorial plaques commemorating in English, Latin and Chinyanja those who died in the service of Likoma. United there were doctors of divinity, deacons and vergers, joiners and masons, black and white.

This commingling was not whimsical: the wildly different components all had meaning. Everything was the product of shared history brought to fruitfulness together; of richness and variety of learning; and of lives given freely to this place.

XXI

INTERLUDE IN ZANZIBAR

'To the glory of God and in memory of Livingstone and other explorers, men good and brave, who, to advance knowledge, set free the slave, and hasten Christ's kingdom in Africa, loved not their lives even unto death.'

So reads the inscription beneath a window in the cathedral in Zanzibar, to where the Universities' Mission to Central Africa had to relocate for a few years when the number of casualties in Malaŵi became insupportable. It was at this headquarters that Maples and Johnson first adjusted to life in Africa; and from here that they set off in the direction of Lake Malaŵi.

The cathedral, constructed on the site of what was then Africa's largest slave-market, was designed so that the altar would occupy the spot where slaves were once tethered to a post and looked in the mouth. Its architects sought to eliminate all traces of the macabre from the place but, by an oversight, they neglected to demolish a single small dungeon from the block across the way which had been used to house slaves. It is into this tiny space, recently embellished by a few rusty chains, that tourists now pack themselves to marvel at the ghastliness. The conditions in which the slaves were kept are brought vividly to life by the lurid descriptions of local tour guides. You have to pay and queue for some time for this experience. It then costs a dollar or two more to enter the cathedral itself.

'Is it actually worth it?' I was asked by a party of Scandinavian NGO workers, as I wandered out of the church. They had already paid for the 'cell experience' but were in two minds about entering what might be the world's greatest monument to abolitionism.

I knew they were NGO workers because I chanced upon them later in a local bar. 'We are humanitarians' was their unabashed answer when I asked them what they did. Theirs was a field project in a remote part of the mainland. They had come to this island paradise for a week of rest and recuperation.

Despite crowds of tourists, Zanzibar is still an enchanted place. It was once the capital of a sprawling Arab empire that arose in Muscat but was re-centred on the east coast of Africa, whence flowed its slaves, gold and spices. As it crumbled, it became the focus of intrigue between competing imperial powers. After a period of German influence, it was absorbed as a British protectorate in 1896, following the shortest war in history: the sultan surrendered after his palace was bombarded for thirty-eight minutes by British gunboats. His successor was installed as a puppet ruler and subdued into abolishing slavery.

The sultans went on, more and more enervated, until overthrown by Marxist revolutionaries in 1964. Their protracted decline has today resulted in one of the world's great conglomerations of fallen grandeur. The town is a mass of comely dereliction, of splendour amid decay that will gratify the deepest *nostalgie de la boue*. Among fallen palaces and dilapidated mosques wind labyrinthine streets, cluttered with refuse. Dirty spires and minarets tower above ornate houses, built tall to block out the sun, even at noon, when the main thoroughfares rejoice in crepuscular gloom.

The rats are fat and nonchalant, wandering unmolested among torpid alley cats.

The quayside is still very much alive, now with the lumbering of dockworkers, the clang of cargo ships, and the whir of light aircraft circling above the port. As the sun sets, the calls of the muezzin rise above the din, and you start to catch the occasional waft of clove and coconut breaking through the familiar, all-pervasive smell of old rubbish. As the warm, smoky evening deepens, the promenade starts to bustle with society, the townsfolk emerging from their worship to wander among the barbecues and confectioners of the night market. Here you feast on fresh crab and lobster fragrantly spiced, on guavas, sherbets and yielding gelatinous puddings.

I watched two corpulent gentlemen in flowing robes exchange elaborate greetings, their retinues waiting patiently behind them, faces and bodies decorously covered. As the two parted company, one noticed that his shoelace had come undone. He snapped his fingers at one of the women, who came forward and knelt before him in the street to re-tie it.

Here in Zanzibar a splendid cosmopolitanism has been achieved, with Arab and African traditions steeped in a myriad of outside influences from the whole basin of the Indian Ocean and beyond. To the Western tourist it seems a delightful entrepôt, even a triumph of cultural exchange. But the integration has been driven by cold impulses: conquest, domination, commercial interest. There is not the atmosphere of curiosity and high learning felt at Likoma. The marks of other cultures are all around you, but they have been imposed, accepted for convenience or embraced out of caprice. The town's great collection is the House of Wonders, a shambling palace made into a cavern of toys and trinkets that the sultans exacted as tribute or otherwise amassed from holidays around the world. Priceless artefacts are juxtaposed with junk: lustrous old ivory surrounds garish chinoiserie, mass-produced in Britain in the nineteenth century. Fine Zanzibari wood-carvings and exquisite Asian lacquerware are offset by dismal oil paintings and tin toys. In one room, you find rare Arab silver and costly Persian rugs; in the next is the last sultan's bidet. It is charming but uninformed, the multiculturalism of the magpie.

And is there not also a flavour of sybaritic cruelty to Zanzibar? It is impossible to ignore the long shadow of slavery. In the handsome, varied features of its peoples, are you witnessing the product of harems only recently closed, into which exotic beauties were cherry-picked from around the world like the trifles in the House of Wonders?

But these concerns seemed distant at the bar where I again encountered the Scandinavians. They were part of a small, relaxed throng of Westerners, mostly other NGO workers on holiday. Their projects were the usual blend of small-scale infrastructure, women's empowerment, microfinance. They expected to stay in Africa for one or two years. Their engagement was fleeting, their curiosity limited. They had gone into the church in the end but emerged underwhelmed and perplexed, and had not noticed the plaque. Of the Universities' Mission they knew nothing, though they had heard of Livingstone. 'They were all just colonialists, right? We're not so interested in that stuff.' They were drinking, playing pool, chatting and flirting at a bar in which the only Africans were staff, weed vendors or prostitutes. The first two groups were doing a good trade, but the last seemed to have given up on finding custom. The Scandinavians were more interested in a couple of Irish girls wearing 'hakuna matata' T-shirts, whom they were teaching how to order a beer in Swahili. They then moved on to discuss a nearby vegan deli, recently opened, and Barack Obama, who was in Nairobi deploring homophobia. I felt stuck in a simulacrum of conversation I had experienced in a dozen other places from London to Bangkok – conversation inevitable where young Westerners gather, impossible where they do not.

I thought of Johnson and Maples, their sacrifice and moral seriousness, their curiosity, solitude and open-mindedness. 'We must lay aside all ideas of being mirrors of the world, and must be servants of those we are meant to serve,' Johnson had asserted. But the final word in Zanzibar went to a British tourist who passed a confused judgement in the cathedral visitors' book: 'Boring. Slavery was created by us – Western barbarism remaining here.'

XXII

IN MEMORIAM

Blantyre, the city named for Livingstone's birthplace, is Malaŵi's commercial capital. There are supermarkets and fast-food joints, a dual carriageway and a scattering of street lamps. Piped water and electricity are supplied, albeit erratically. It is hard to imagine it other than as a modern city, with an educated middle class and plenty of expatriates, often seen jogging up and down its hills in Fitbits and Lycra, past locals trudging under their usual hefty burdens. But Blantyre's claim to urban sophistication was undermined in 2017 when the city made international news because of a vampire crisis.

Blood-sucking supernatural beings were first sighted in the countryside further south but then started to predate on city folk. In the ensuing panic, people were killed on suspicion of being vampires or their accomplices. As the death toll rose well into double figures, NGOs and aid organisations, including the Red Cross, were evacuated from the worst affected areas. There remains as of yet no definite end to or explanation for the affair. When I last visited, expatriate life in the city seemed keen to move on from this small eruption of the primordial out of the surface of gentility.

None of this would have surprised David Clement Scott, who arrived in Blantyre to lead the mission there in 1881 when it was just a tiny island of European settlement in an ocean of bush. Over the next seventeen years, Scott made Malaŵi's indigenous culture the object of passionate study, defying the suspicion this aroused in fellow Europeans. Vampires and other ghouls are encompassed with equanimity in his book, his descriptions suggesting they have changed little over the last hundred years.

Blantyre is high up on top of a vertiginous escarpment, amid the cool, fertile undulations of the Shire Highlands. Far below – though only a few miles as the crow flies – extends a torrid, malarial flatland that drains into the Zambezi basin. Livingstone led a disastrous expedition here in 1863, which failed in all its objectives and sustained heavy casualties. Two young Englishmen expired together of dysentery at the very foot of the escarpment, gazing up helplessly at the salubrious heights just beyond their reach. 'Ye shall be witnesses unto me' is the epitaph on one of the tombstones; 'Where I am, there shall also my servant be' reads the other. The graves are in a lonely, stifling place but are honoured today nevertheless.

The Church of Scotland persisted in the area despite the failure of that expedition. Thanks to a coincidence of commercial interests, its mission at Blantyre was well established when Scott was appointed to lead it, but he arrived in the wake of scandal. His predecessor, it emerged, had been presiding over a cruel and incompetent tyranny: lashings had become normalised, and two Africans had been sentenced to death. One turned out to be innocent, the other executed so clumsily that the method amounted to torture.

In Scott, the mission could scarcely have found a gentler replacement. A native of Edinburgh, middle-class and educated in Classics and mathematics, he was a sensitive man, delicate in mind and body, a lover of languages, poetry and music. His slight form was only accentuated by a furious Nietzschean moustache, and a glint in his eye hinted at a capacity for wild obsession. The violence and misrule ceased, and Scott threw himself into everything with a rapturous amateur spirit. He preached, travelled and taught, attempting an ambitious and holistic curriculum that encompassed arts and sciences. 'Hebrew lessons are finally starting this month!' he writes with child-like glee in the mission chronicle.

'His mind and soul dwelt among the higher entities of life', yet Scott was 'not unpractical', observed a friend. In the centre of Blantyre, he designed and built a huge and elaborate church, though his experience in architecture and engineering was nil. From its complexity – Byzantine dome, giddy towers and elaborate woodwork (which Scott carved himself) – you derive strong intimations of its designer's eccentricity.

However, Scott's greatest achievements were in his study of the languages and culture of the local people – in particular, his *Cyclopaedic Dictionary of the Mang'anja Language*. It is the work of a gifted and rigorous linguist, a painstaking study of vocabulary, grammar, syntax and phonology. By applying the philological equipment he had acquired from studying ancient languages at university, he achieved a systematic ordering of every detail of Mang'anja, from palatals to plosives, prefixes and pronominal particles.

The dictionary was also 'cyclopaedic'. Almost every entry includes an (often lengthy) contextual account of the word being defined, and so the whole becomes a treasure-house of Scott's accumulated knowledge of the indigenous culture. This knowledge was diverse because he was enraptured by everything he encountered: he came to know the people's customs in life and death, their gods and their spirits; he learnt their crafts, from pottery and weaving to growing and fishing, construction of huts and of traps, the secrets of hunter and herbalist. He delighted in all the country's manifestations of life, down to its grasses and insects. He even enthused about the local cuisine, which he describes with unexpected relish. He may be the first European to have reported a fondness for maize porridge, the country's unlovely national dish.

Scott was also able to relate his findings to the aspects of his own culture that he loved most. Like Johnson, he 'found affinities' everywhere he looked. In Mang'anja's accidence, inflections and verbal reduplications, he heard familiar echoes of classical languages and Hebrew. In the rhythms of its speech, he detected the metrical effects of Horace's Latin verse. He compared its stories to the mythology of Greece. And he heaped praises on its music, integrating native song with Gregorian chant in his own compositions.

David Clement Scott was besotted with the country, so much so that you encounter him bending over backwards to excuse what most would condemn. He defended rain prayers when most missionaries were wary of sanctioning superstition: 'It is not fetish, it is a purely natural religion with the religious element left in, just as Comtism leaves it out,' he pronounced archly. Any imputation of savagery seemed to stir a prickly defensiveness. That suspected witches were burnt and poisoned, he could not deny, but his reflex was to snap back at any assertion of superiority: how long ago was it that we in Europe stopped doing the same? You even encounter an awkward tone of special pleading as he tries to explain away the practice of hurling slaves and widows into the grave with the departed chief. The practice was rare, dying out and, anyway, had only ever been reserved for special occasions, he explained meekly.

It was in the sphere of language that Scott's infatuation was wildest. The dictionary is for the most part a work of serious academic endeavour, an ordering of every aspect of Mang'anja into the strict categories of the philologist. In its introduction, however, Scott gives free rein to his rhapsodic tendencies and declares love. Mang'anja, he proclaims, possesses the fullest expression of the abstract yet achieved by man, and reaches closer than any other tongue to the breath of God. For page after lyrical page of fanciful linguistic theorising, he claims its superiority in spiritual force to any other language he knew – and he knew many.

> What strikes one born in all the formulas of civilisation [. . .] which, like a veil, conceal the vision of truth, is the living touch of the Bantu speech with its root ideas. It speaks from nature, but it speaks from God. It is the witness of a perfect incarnation [. . .] And any who would surpass it must be as broad and courteous as this language and this people declare the genius of Africa to be.

'God forbid that I should presume to understand him!' commented a friend and colleague at the Blantyre mission. Scott was a baffling man, and I am certainly not qualified to pass judgement on his linguistic theories, but what is absolutely clear is the sincerity of his esteem for the language and culture in which he immersed himself.

Unfortunately Scott found that education was indivisible from politics, even or especially when its goals were loftiest. He was adamant that more responsibility for leadership should be handed to Africans and worked closely with seven Malawian deacons whom he ordained and instructed. But Scott's mission was at the heart of a fast-growing stronghold of white settlement. He and the landowners soon came to blows.

'The land is not ours to begin with,' Scott ventured quixotically. 'We cannot treat the natives as a conquered race [. . .] They accorded us permission to dwell among them [. . .] and every planter in the country has entered into the privileges he possesses under this missionary attitude and promise.'

The white planters would hear none of it and engineered a campaign of petty persecution and undermining. After a relentless two years – during which his wife, brother and young son all died of fever – Scott's spirits were broken, and he allowed himself to be driven from the Blantyre Mission by his settler enemies. He took up an obscure position in Kenya, where he was soon after laid to rest. He has now vanished into near total obscurity, a quiet martyr to the cause of open-mindedness.

XXIII

LIVINGSTONIA

The north of Malaŵi is dominated by a vast desolate plateau of over a thousand square miles. It is almost untouched by human habitation and might be the setting for Conan Doyle's *Lost World*. Its edges are sheer and rocky, but, on its surface, you find yourself among gently rolling hills and shimmering grassland, seemingly without end. Dusk transforms all into a ghostly, lunar landscape; the air grows cold, and leopards emerge from patches of forest to lay uncontested claim to the immense territory.

At the plateau's eastern edge, foothills rise abruptly out of Lake Malaŵi, and ascent looks impossible. Even today, getting there is a challenging drive up the Gorodi Road, a rough dirt track that climbs 2,000 feet in three miles. After twenty-two memorable hairpin bends, you are astonished to arrive at what resembles a small Scottish town, with terraced houses, cathedral and a university – all poised like a lonely eyrie over the Great Rift Valley. This is Livingstonia, a settlement and educational project of soaring ambition, and the vision of one man: Dr Robert Laws. In Britain today, his name has vanished into the obscurity from which it emerged, but this titan of the Victorian age is still remembered as a hero in Malaŵi.

Laws was born in 1851 to an Aberdeen cabinet-maker in whose craft he became a keen and industrious apprentice.

He had a prodigious mind and, like his hero Livingstone, taught himself Classics, theology and the sciences in rare moments spared from toil. His family were poor, and he handed over much of his weekly salary to help his stepmother run the household. With what he could save, he bought books. A Greek grammar which he coveted was beyond his means, so he prevailed on the bookseller to let him borrow it, and then reproduced a complete copy for himself by hand. After years of evening classes and laborious self-education, he was admitted to the University of Aberdeen, where he took degrees in both arts and medicine. He then enrolled to train as a medical missionary, determined to follow in Livingstone's footsteps in Africa. On qualifying, he stubbornly resisted efforts to have him sent elsewhere, and in 1875 was dispatched to what is now Malaŵi.

The Anglicans, under Maples and Johnson, were already dying in droves on the eastern side of the lake. For a while, on the opposite shore, the Scottish Presbyterian Mission added to the death toll, and Laws was driven from station to station as each had to be abandoned to malaria. After five years of graves and failures, he settled on a radical solution: he would relocate to an austere mountain fastness, high above the tropical miasma of the flatland.

The construction of Livingstonia was an heroic endeavour, and Laws appears as a figure of almost mythological greatness. His gigantic frame and luxuriant beard recall Hellenistic depictions of Hercules, and he laboured at everything, impelled by a dour puritanical commitment to exhaust both mind and body every day except the Sabbath. He worked alongside the African labourers at road-building, brick-moulding, lime-firing, stone-cutting, ploughing and planting. Church and houses, workshops, schools and a hospital went up, and Laws received the morass of diseased humanity into his clinics and operating theatre. He then thundered from the pulpit before whirling from cowshed to quarry, from sawmill to smithy, demonstrating all he knew of carpentry and metalwork, masonry and animal husbandry.

Laws had chosen a hostile part of Malaŵi, where many locals were from tribes terrorised by slavers and the Ngoni. But he was undeterred, and the mission sent two other formidable Scotsmen to live among the warrior peoples and urge them to peace. Laws meanwhile won prestige when, unarmed, he berated a party of slavers so furiously that they surrendered their caravan without a fight. On another occasion, he was mauled by a lion but fended it off with his bare hands. And when the Germans invaded from Tanganyika in 1914, reaching perilously close to Livingstonia, his instructions to the mission were in the high tradition of the British stiff upper lip: 'Sit tight, allay panic, continue work as usual.' The Germans were duly repelled.

As the settlement grew, Laws turned his hand to engineering, laying five miles of pipe to make Livingstonia the first town in the region to enjoy running water. Then he set his mind to electricity, still a rarity back in Britain. Teaching himself the principles of electrical engineering, he began work on a small hydroelectric power station, and by 1905 he had it up and running. It was the first attempt to generate electricity on a large scale anywhere in the country, and even today provides Livingstonia with a more reliable supply than that enjoyed by the rest of Malaŵi, every other district of which knows almost daily power cuts.

From the start, everything had to go up the mountain, even before a cart or pack animals could manage the route. Cubes of granite, miles of cable, lengths of pipe, telegraph wire, pylons, generator, the church's mighty brass lectern –

all went up that terrible road. Among the very first items to ascend were a steel printing press and – shortly afterwards – a second, even larger one.

The presses were prioritised, because, from the start, Laws intended the highest educational endeavour, with arts and letters central to his vision. He had acquired several local languages himself, beginning by dauntlessly pointing to a tree and noting down the name the locals gave for it. After eight years, his mastery was such that not only had he produced a translation of the New Testament, he had taught his parishioners to read it.

At first, the local population had consisted of herders and warriors, all illiterate. At Livingstonia, they learnt letters, numeracy and scripture but also all the practical skills required to run this modern, functioning town. Still Laws wanted more, and he began to develop a curriculum of almost unlimited scope. This was offered at the Overtoun Institute, founded at Livingstonia in 1894 and named for one of the mission's most generous Scottish donors. Here, the brightest students had the opportunity to study literature, history, philosophy, theology, Latin, Ancient Greek and Hebrew. Indeed for a motto, Laws turned to Greek: πειράσω – 'I will try.'

'Compare and contrast the moral philosophies of Plato and Aristotle.'

'Distinguish Trinity from Tri-Unity.'

'God does not by predestination destroy that freedom in me which is essential to moral growth. Discuss.'

These were exam questions which Malaŵian students had to answer to graduate from the Overtoun Institute – and answer them they did.

The results were spectacular. After twelve years, this warlike region had been entirely pacified without a shot being fired. Thirty-three thousand students had passed through the Institute, and a thousand new master craftsmen had been trained. By 1934, when Laws died at the age of eighty-three, the north of Malaŵi was claimed to be the most literate and educationally developed province of any country in British Africa. From Livingstonia's printing presses rolled off translations of the gospels into twelve native languages. From its poets and musicians came vernacular hymnals. And from among the brightest graduates came pastors, teachers, writers and thinkers – learned men and women, independent in mind and spirit. To note just a few:

Clements Kadalie left Malaŵi for South Africa, where he became a founder member of the ANC, an important enemy of apartheid, and Africa's most distinguished trade unionist.

Yesaya Mwase was among Laws' ablest students of Latin and Greek. He became one of the first three pastors to be ordained from Livingstonia and went on to found his own independent black church – as did his fellow graduates, Charles Domingo and Yafet Mkandawire.

Charles Chinula became a successful opponent of unjust colonial policy, while also translating Bunyan's *Pilgrim's Progress* and Shakespeare's *Julius Caesar* into native languages – projects sponsored financially by Kamuzu Banda from the proceeds of his medical practice in Britain.

David and Helen Kaunda met as students at Livingstonia. Both became professional teachers and were the parents of the late Kenneth Kaunda, who led Zambia to independence and beyond.

Lastly – a few decades later – Legson Kayira graduated from Livingstonia before setting off on foot for America to seek his fortune. He became a successful novelist, but he also wrote an autobiography, in which he identified Robert Laws, Kamuzu Banda and John Bunyan as the inspirations for his remarkable journey. Kayira called the book *I Will Try* – after Laws' motto.

The efforts of Livingstonia were supported by the colonial authorities. Indeed, their encouragement made it a victim of its own success, as the abundant supply of educated young men was diverted out of Malaŵi to feed the demand for clerks and managers in the booming industries of South Africa and the Rhodesias – a disastrous prototype of the 'brain drain' phenomenon that is observed in so much of Africa today.

But the proliferation of intelligent critics of imperial rule also became problematic for the government. A commission was set up to examine the whole purpose of education in Africa. Its conclusions were divisive and curiously anticipate many educational controversies in Britain today.

Laws' vision was condemned as pointless extravagance: teaching Latin and Greek, history and literature was wasteful. What possible justification could there be for lavishing resources on academic luxuries when there was an entire country to be trained in more useful, basic vocational skills? The goal should be 'to produce good, contented and loyal African citizens'.

One of Laws' supporters, Donald Fraser, retorted that the purpose of education should sometimes be to produce *discontented* people as well. But that view became suddenly very unpopular in 1915 when an educated Malaŵian pastor, John Chilembwe, who had set up his own mission station, incited his congregation to rebel against British rule. A Livingstonia graduate, George Mwase, later wrote a eulogistic account of this, in which he imagined Chilembwe leading his followers into battle with rousing speeches studded with Latin quotation.

The rebellion petered out after a few days, having failed to attract any popular support. Decades later, Chilembwe would be reinvented as a Malaŵian patriotic hero. At the time, however, the only real effect of his rebellion was to stiffen settler opposition against Laws and his ilk, who were condemned for being hell-bent on over-educating Africans.

Laws' response was combative: the rebellion was 'proof of the need for more, not less education for Africans'. That education should never be compromised, he insisted. 'To discard or even lessen the literary training would be to block the way for advancement of native leaders and means the reduction of the natives to a class of helots.'

The wrangling continued, but, in the end, the technocrats had their way, without upholding or repudiating either principle in the debate. A cost-benefit analysis deemed the exaltation of Laws' vision to be unsustainable, and it was whittled down to something resembling a compromise from which it never recovered. It is unsurprising that this should later have been lamented by Banda, in whose vision you also detect the long influence of Livingstonia. 'Without the Church of Scotland, there would be no Malaŵi,' he declared emphatically. And when he spoke of his own youthful intellectual ambitions, his words might have been those of Robert Laws: 'You may be trained as a doctor, but to be educated is something else – and I wanted to be educated.'

However, debasing the curriculum would never get the genie of political consciousness back into the bottle; independence was less than a generation away. Indeed, several Livingstonia graduates paved the way for Banda's return to Malaŵi, and the membership of the country's first political party, the Nyasaland African Congress, was initially drawn almost wholesale from Livingstonia's debating and literary societies.

It is no surprise, then, that the Northern Region was the focus of crisis and consternation as British rule came to an end. On the lakeshore below the plateau, a state of emergency was triggered in 1958 when colonial troops opened fire on a rioting mob. The white population was fearful of reprisals, and the RAF flew low over Livingstonia, dropping a message from their plane. Was the mission in danger? Should troops be sent to facilitate an evacuation? The aircraft would fly past at the same time the following day to look for an answer marked on the ground.

Outside the church, the mission staff arranged shiny white stones on the grass. When the pilots returned, they found that these read: *EPH. 2.14*. They turned back to base where they looked up the reference in Saint Paul's *Epistle to the Ephesians*. Within days, the mission's avowal of goodwill and racial harmony was on the front page of *The Times* of London: 'For he is our peace, who hath made both one, and hath broken down the middle wall of partition between us.'

No troops were needed at Livingstonia. Life at the mission continued, the state of emergency passed, and the authorities started planning for independence.

There are similarities between Laws and Albert Schweitzer, the Franco-German doctor and philanthropist who won far greater acclaim, even a Nobel Peace Prize, for his labours deep in French West Africa. But their outlooks were different, and Schweitzer's mission hospital at Lambarene never had the educational vision of Livingstonia. Indeed, visitors were shocked at how little effort went into training locals, so that even in the 1960s all the nurses were still volunteers from Europe.

'The African is my brother, it is true – but my junior brother,' Schweitzer infamously asserted. Laws could be paternalistic too, but not with the negativity you sometimes encounter in Schweitzer: 'I put a mango here, a banana here, a breadfruit here,' he once grumbled. 'The Africans do not know enough to tell which tree is which. I explain. They walk away and by the time they reach the river in ten minutes they have forgotten.'

By contrast, Laws maintained an unshakeable faith in the high possibilities of education in Africa. Its goal was nothing less than 'the coordination of technical and literary training to fit the individual to make the most of his life for the service of God, for his own good, and for the good of his fellow men'.

When he taught furniture-making, his own and his father's craft, he was noted to be obsessive in the attention to detail he demanded of his apprentices. Colleagues complained that there was no need to teach Africans to produce elaborate inlays or delicate fretwork. But Laws insisted that the finest possible work must always be the ambition.

His house at Livingstonia reveals the same mentality. It was the first building in Malaŵi to be built of stone, using massive squares of rock hewn from a quarry on the plateau and hauled over to the mission. He refused to economise on the thickness of the walls, which had all to be of top-grade dressed ashlar. And so it was while he was away on a trip that another missionary quickly put on the roof so that Laws could not go through with his original plan to construct another storey. The result is something resembling a modest Scottish manor house, possessing simple elegance and solidity rather than grandeur. From its steps you look out over a small rose garden, then a sheer drop towards the immense lake far below.

As he explained to his wife, before she committed to be his companion of fifty years in Africa, 'You will not be going to live in a mud hut and eat off enamel plates. God does not want your grave, he wants your work – your best work.' Laws saw it as right that he should live in relative dignity and comfort, but the house is far from luxurious. The couple were clearly Spartan in their practices, and there is a draughty Highland atmosphere to the place.

What the house was really designed to show off was a principle – that of doing everything to the highest possible standard. He had a contempt for meanness, for any impulse to scrimp, not because he loved extravagance, but because he rejoiced in what was fulsome and excellent. He extended this to everything he did in Malaŵi, but especially to education. Others argued for the lowest common denominator, for the bare minimum only to be attempted. Laws was convinced that Africans should have access to what he called 'the whole mass of man's spiritual treasures'.

A few years after Laws' death in 1934, the English anthropologist Margaret Read was sent from SOAS to study the tribes of northern Malaŵi. One day she was surprised to be accosted in the wilderness by a young Ngoni warrior brandishing a book: 'You know this book is all about the kind of things we talk about in our village,' he announced. 'This man has wisdom – the kind of wisdom our fathers have. Has he written any other books?' she was asked. It was a copy of Plato's *Republic*.

XXIV

ANCIENT & MODERN

Mua Mission lies amid sultry woodland in the foothills of the Dedza Highlands. At its boundary, you can look down on a deep, narrow gorge sundered by prehistoric forces. From the stream below are said to rise tutelary water sprites who protect the community and vouchsafe rains. There is a numinous atmosphere to the place, and even my most skeptical friends have felt unsettled by the peculiar cast of shadows among the trees at dusk, by strange stirrings in the night, by a pentagram of twigs left beside a path.

The mission itself is a fine building, with a loggia framed by Romanesque arches from which you can observe the lake through mists in the far distance; however, it is the museum that best repays attention. It is the work of Claude Boucher, a French-Canadian Catholic missionary who came to the country in the 1960s and has resolutely Malaŵianised. At Mua, he found himself at the meeting point of three tribes: the Chewa, the Ngoni and the Yao. Boucher has studied them all, learning their languages and assimilating a little of each. But it is into the Chewa that he was formally received, accepting the tribal cognomen Chisale and undergoing initiation into the Nyau – perhaps the only Westerner, and surely the only Christian missionary, ever to have done so.

It is this intimacy with the local peoples that has allowed him to amass and explain the contents of the museum. It is above all a celebration of *gule wamkulu*, and the fabulous beasts of the Great Dance erupt from the centre of the main exhibition hall in a cascade of masks and costumes, arranged to imitate the burgeoning of the tree of life. Boucher, who has written an authoritative compendium of the characters of *gule*, here displays the greatest collection of Nyau masks anywhere exhibited.

There is not the sense you get in many museums, of dead artefacts hoovered up from afar and transplanted to a lifeless glass case. The collection is personal and rooted firmly in the place. Boucher's own photographs smother the walls and capture the exhibits alive and in use, recently and nearby: craftsmen and farmers at work with their tools, physicians and diviners meddling with herbs and charms, heavily armed warriors, and chiefs clad in leopard skins presiding over rites of passage. It is a life's labour, a triumph of patience, not only in waiting for rare occasions to present themselves, but also in building the trust needed to secure admission to the most hallowed inner life of the tribes.

A chief has died, and all the rituals of lamentation are captured by Boucher's lens: the keening and the tears, the besmirching of face and body, the tearing of hair and the beating of breasts. The stiffened corpse sits upright in a corner of the room as the family go about their business despite its staring presence. The head is crowned with the intestines of a bull; the inflated bladder affixed to its forehead. And then it is lowered onto a seat in the grave as the last rites of the Church are commingled with more ancient oblations.

Boucher, Scott, Laws and Johnson were extraordinary men, and it cannot be claimed that their examples are typical of all missionaries in Malaŵi. Others were often dismissive if not actively hostile to the indigenous culture. The murderous injustice at the Blantyre Mission before

Scott arrived was exceptional, but common enough was the impulse to suppress 'savage practices', to uproot and destroy anything local. In fact, Banda took as the basis for his own distinction between good and bad missionaries whether or not they celebrated or despised the customs of the place.

Even where there was not revulsion and contempt, there was a good deal of plodding, incurious piety and generally colourless thinking. The historian of the lake, Oliver Ransford, describes the 'awful accumulation of cant' that characterised many of the more workaday missionaries: 'They part from each other "with eyes not dry"; their experiences are always "the reverse of disappointing" [. . .] They rarely travel as ordinary people do but "pass by on their Master's business" [. . .] Native customs that might shock the laity are either ignored or concealed [. . .] and we are not surprised that their own trousers are termed "unmentionables".'

At first the Catholics were as eager as any to extirpate 'sad manifestation of false religion', but, more recently, they have been pre-eminent in defence of local culture. Boucher's late contemporary, Matthew Schoffeleers, became a leading authority on the mythology and pre-Christian religion of Malaŵi; Boucher himself regularly appears on Malaŵian TV to lament and warn against the neglect of ancient knowledge. His own mass is a triumph of syncretism which, before the licence of the Second Vatican Council, might have necessitated a break with Rome.

In vestments of black and orange, the celebrants advance down the nave, followed by book and thurible. Behind them throng dancing girls, with leaps, bounds and shrill ululation. All are clad in commemorative *chitenjes* printed in blue and orange with the face of their new boy king. A leopard's skin is draped on the altar and the congregation is summoned to prayer. Hands are raised to the sky in an ambiguous gesture of thanks and supplication, and fingers quiver as arms descend in imitation and invocation of falling rain. The key moments from the mass are unmistakable, but much is deeply obscure, as when a large round plastic mirror is paraded before the tabernacle. Next, the congregation breaks into a hymn of thanksgiving as an offertory procession advances up the nave. To the slow beat of drums, their simple gifts are carried forward: small parcels of rice, sugar or eggs, a bundle of potatoes, a single large pawpaw. These are the gifts of the very poor, borne with pride towards the altar in a dignified, lilting step. The host is immolated with maize flour and the pink and white petals of bougainvillea. Then the priest elevates the bread and wine, as the audience stare fixedly at the magic of transubstantiation.

After the service, a small throng gathers around Boucher, to whom Chichewa now comes more readily than English, as he discourses on land disputes and bad weather, a local scandal and intrigues at the court of the new king who, until his coronation, was being taught Latin by Dr Highbrow. His stories abound with the ongoing machinations of devious chiefs and jealous queens – incomprehensible to anyone not involved. Scott, Laws and Johnson had in common a spirit of total immersion in the world around them, of warm and abiding commitment to the place. The same is obvious in Boucher as he rambles on, lost to his obscure and subtle theme, working through an endless succession of mentholated cigarettes.

However, the traditional churches – Catholic, Anglican, Presbyterian – are shrinking in Malaŵi, losing their congregations to evangelical newcomers. These originate mostly from America and arrive in droves, many impelled by Behemoth financial endowments and corporate mission statements. One or two have constructed sprawling headquarters in Malaŵi's capital, gargantuan structures gleaming with newly imported building materials. Their names often struck me as outlandish, but I suspect a litigious tendency and so will clump them under the designation favoured by Dr Highbrow: the Quivering Brethren.

My first encounters with the Quivering Brethren were in the high-end supermarkets of Lilongwe and Blantyre when, standing in the queue, I found myself elbowed by a clutch of pale-faced, busy-looking young Americans in short-sleeved shirts buttoned primly to the top. As they earnestly unloaded mountains of soft drinks and salty snacks from their shopping trolleys, they avoided eye contact and engaged only cursorily with the checkout girl, preferring to talk surreptitiously among themselves.

Over time, I noticed that trips to the capital were rare when I did not spot these tight-knit little groups, usually getting into or out of the largest and shiniest of 4x4 vehicles, emblazoned with the name of the Quivering Brethren and a highly stylised cross.

I noticed their insignia elsewhere, on buildings and ordinary passenger vehicles, which sometimes bore bumper sticker with slogans like 'This Car is Protected by the Blood of Jesus Christ!' or perhaps still more alarmingly 'Bathed in the Blood of the Lamb!'

The Quivering Brethren concentrated their efforts in the cities, but converts scattered widely, among rich and poor alike. Flemings' family had been Anglicans for as long as anyone could remember, so when his son Harvey joined the Quivering Brethren, there was considerable discord.

'In my life I was not doing well,' he explained when I met him in Blantyre. But since switching churches he had found a job and now worked at a mini-mart owned by another member of the congregation. 'To what do you attribute your success?' he asked me disarmingly. To deflect the question, I wondered if I might join him for one of his church's services, and Harvey gladly agreed.

Held in a small breeze-block hall in a poor suburb, the service was so loud we could hear it from some distance as we approached. We entered halfway through, as a Malaŵian preacher in a natty suit assailed the congregation through a microphone. Its members were being singled out and wildly applauded, for securing new jobs, pay rises or otherwise meeting with good fortune. My understanding was mediated through Harvey's translations, but the victories seemed to be rather of the flesh than the spirit, with prosperity attributed to the love of Jesus Christ, directed onto them by the Church of the Quivering Brethren. At one point there was a salacious exchange about a Mercedes-Benz.

At Boucher's mass, there had been something free and vital in the participation of those present. Here, I felt as if I were watching a demonstration of mesmerism. I was the only foreigner present, and the pastor kept catching my eye as he scanned the crowd. I began to fear that my skepticism was somehow plainly visible, especially when he pronounced in English: 'Jesus loves all of *you*!' while staring accusingly at me. I never imagined those words could be intoned so menacingly. I decided to slip out in the middle of a jingling evangelical hymn.

The Quivering Brethren seemed inescapable. When I later returned to Malaŵi as a doctor, I frequently found them waiting outside the entrance to the big city hospital where I was working. One day I asked them what they were doing, but they seemed disinclined to speak to me, answering guardedly that they were just there to offer help and comfort to anyone who needed it. One of the Malaŵian nurses was censorious, explaining to me that they were there to recruit patients and their relatives, hoping to find them receptive in an hour of distress or extremity.

And then atop a mountain plateau, I encountered a whole party of adolescent Brethren out hiking, supervised by a red-faced American and a local Malaŵian pastor in wrap-around sunglasses. The youths were all white Americans and were quite voluble when I spoke to them, although the two adults eyed me warily. They were on a teen evangelical mission, touring seven African countries in six weeks, and were paying the Quivering Brethren for the opportunity to do so.

On the good news that they claimed to be spreading, I cannot comment. But there seemed little possibility on a trip like that of the sort of engagement achieved by Johnson, Scott, Laws or Boucher in the course of their long careers in Africa. Those men's starting point had been humility, which seemed in short supply here.

'We've come to proclaim and magnify the truth of Lord Jesus,' stated the leader of the group matter-of-factly. 'We've just done South Africa, Zimbabwe and Zambia. After Malaŵi, we're doing Tanzania, Uganda and Kenya.'

I wished them well and inwardly hoped they possessed even a little of the sensibility of David Clement Scott. 'Africa is an education,' he had asserted. 'Here you come to school again. In this new school of service, we must learn before we can teach.'

XXV

DEA EX MACHINA

One day I happened to join a colleague on her visit to a rural orphanage. Several other Westerners were in the party, and we were welcomed excitedly by the Malaŵian pastor in charge of the foundation, which was supported by the Quivering Brethren.

He explained, over the course of a long sermon, that he was not surprised to see us there – we had been sent by God. He knew this because the orphanage was again in need of funds, and so he had recently 'faxed' God a message to ask for assistance. Now He had provided. Afterwards we were taken outside on a tour, during which excited children tussled with each other to attract our attention. Eventually we were led up behind the orphanage onto high ground, where a small brick hut nestled among trees. This, the pastor explained, was where his prayers were offered, and answered. Indeed, according to a boldly painted sign, here was 'The Fax Machine to God'.

The effectiveness of this means of appeal was firmly established. For once, when the orphanage had been in direst need, God had responded to the pastor's fax with generosity beyond anyone's wildest dreams: he had sent Madonna.

The American popular musician has had a special interest in Malaŵi for a number of years. Her estimated personal wealth is a substantial fraction of the country's entire GDP, and she has generously supported schools, orphanages, clinics and a miscellany of other development projects. She has also added four Malaŵian children to her family, which already consisted of a biological son and daughter, by different fathers. The first Malaŵian child was adopted in 2006, after a mutually satisfactory arrangement was reached with the boy's father, a subsistence farmer. Two years later, Madonna identified an orphaned girl recovering in hospital from meningitis. She cradled the child in her arms, and, as with David, reportedly promised to take her into her family before she had any legal guarantee that this would be possible. Indeed, the Malaŵian judiciary rejected her application to adopt, pointing to the complicated domestic circumstances in which her family already lived. Madonna was undeterred: 'You can imagine how I received this information. It's true, I am a freedom fighter. I am a feminist. I am a rebel heart. But I am also a compassionate and intelligent human being. And if you cannot give me a logical reason for the word "no", then I will not accept the word "no". I hired a team of lawyers, and I took my case to the supreme court.'

Malaŵi's adoption laws 'had not been reformed since the early '40s, and it had not occurred to anyone to change them yet', she averred. The government would shortly take deep offence at her high-handed, even minatory tone. But Madonna did get her way, following a legal wrangle and – it was reported – the distribution of bounteous largesse. 'Love conquers all,' she proclaimed.

Madonna visits Malaŵi frequently, often booking out an entire luxury resort in the capital to guarantee her privacy. From there she is shuttled to her various projects around the country. In the course of one of these trips, she fell out with the then President Joyce Banda (no relation of Kamuzu

– Banda is a common name), to whom she had suggested a meeting, in a strange, over-familiar note penned on her arrival at Lilongwe airport. Banda declined the invitation, and Madonna left disappointed, later complaining of the insult of having to go through normal airport check-in and security.

There followed a bold public statement from the president, who accused Madonna of bullying local officials and exaggerating her philanthropy. It was 'strange and depressing', she observed, 'that Madonna wants Malaŵi to be forever chained to the obligation of gratitude. [. . .] If [kindness] can't be free and silent, it is not kindness; it is something else. Blackmail is the closest it becomes.'

But Joyce Banda soon fell amid scandals of her own, and her successor warmly endorsed Madonna after she increased her donations to become Malaŵi's biggest individual benefactor. Her generosity even extended to a children's hospital, named after her daughter.

Madonna then set about expanding her family further, this time by adopting twins. There were more legal obstacles to overcome and, in the course of the hearing, Madonna's motivation and ability to care for the children was scrutinised. Her legal team thought it relevant to draw the court's attention to the fact that Madonna's natural daughter has her adoptive sister's name tattooed on her arm, and that her adoptive son, David, had expressed a desire to become President of Malaŵi (an ambition Madonna has celebrated on social media).

There was an attempt to uphold the normal legal requirement of eighteen months' residence in Malaŵi on the part of the prospective parent, during which time the relationship could be assessed by the authorities. But in the end this was overlooked, and Madonna, who often stays only a few days at a time in Malaŵi, returned to Europe with the twins in her private jet.

Since then, the press has reported on unedifying squabbles with the families of all Madonna's adoptive children, only one of whom was in fact parentless, for the status of orphanhood is complicated in Malaŵi. The predominant Chewa tribe traditionally observe matrilineal descent and allow children to be raised by the mother's extended family rather than by both parents. Recourse to 'orphanages' for support is a common occurrence but is often only a temporary arrangement in periods of hardship. In any given orphanage, few residents may actually be true orphans.

Regardless, Madonna was granted the right to adopt because this was judged to be in the best interests of the children in question. On one level, it was an easy choice: a life of privilege and unlimited wealth, or one of great insecurity and probable hardship. But there was much that the court, with its necessarily narrow focus on the welfare of particular children, could not consider: the licence and encouragement that the judgement might give to others; the implied reduction of Malaŵian children to the status of commodities for Westerners with buying power; the potential harm to the country's own honourable tradition of adoption within the extended family.

Above all, the court could not consider all the children who do not get chosen. For these, the psychological effect of witnessing adoption by Madonna might be powerfully demoralising. If you live in poverty and then see your peers exalted by a *dea ex machina* to a life of joyful plenty, your own possibilities for fulfilment appear shabby by contrast.

Even for the few who *are* chosen, material benefit must somehow be weighed against the intangible and unquantifiable. When Madonna's children arrived in the UK, British social services pointed out the need to 'reinforce the child's ethnic and cultural heritage', but how – practically – do you do this, beyond mere gesturing?

Other American A-listers wander the globe, adopting a Cambodian child here, an Eritrean there, the choice seemingly constrained by fashion: children from, for example, Chad or England are apparently less desirable in Hollywood. Madonna, to her credit, has shown consistency and concentrated her attention on one country.

Several times a year, her children are flown to Malaŵi for holidays and paraded as local celebrities, during which time pictures appear on social media of adventures clad in native costume. But it can look like raiding the dressing-up box, as when Madonna's son was dropped off in the country for a few days so he could attend a village ceremony to receive his tribal name. Can such a custom still be meaningful when its context has been so distorted? Can you properly participate in the course of a flying visit? Perhaps the answer is yes; but there is a danger of grasping only the cosmetic and of trivialising a real culture.

In another photo posted to the world on Twitter, Madonna showed off her son wearing what was supposed to be traditional attire. But it was a woman's dress, and it had been draped stylishly over his shoulder in a way that would never be seen on a boy in Malaŵi. The whole ensemble was offset by a tastefully simple 'ethnic' necklace. It is the tribal wear of the catwalk. 'Be proud of who you are and where you come from' was Madonna's caption to this image of her son.

And what of Madonna's own culture? Bling appears central to the aesthetic in which her children are raised: David and his mother posed at the Grammy Awards in matching Ralph Lauren gangster outfits and, shortly after this, Madonna bought him a set of gold 'teeth grills' to match her own. More recently, three of the children, dressed head-to-toe in matching Gucci tracksuits, have been shown off to journalists. You can marvel at the many levels of irony contained in Madonna's famous self-avowal as 'a material girl in a material world', but there may also be important truth in the statement if taken at face value. Perhaps the countless homes and the private jet are to be expected. But the list of Madonna's dressing-room essentials, diligently catalogued by her fans, reads like a parody of shallow luxury: white roses and a love seat, a Dead Sea foot spa and an oxygen facial machine, unsalted edamame beans and all the smells, bells and candles needed for esoteric devotion.

For Madonna is, or at least was, among the famous adherents of the Kabbalah Centre in New York, which has been described as an expensive, modern cult that invites belief in charms and astrology, hefty donation and the spiritual benefits of certain sexual positions over others. Madonna's children were seen being led into its monumental headquarters in New York, and the centre has involved itself in projects in Malaŵi through Madonna's mediation.

Unease with her own heritage has been a prominent feature of Madonna's art. Raised a Catholic, she famously acted out the crucifixion on stage, being raised on the cross wearing a crown of thorns beside images of Hitler and George Bush. Elsewhere, she has portrayed herself dreaming of sex with a black saint whom she has helped escape from being lynched by the KKK, whose crosses burn in the background as she develops stigmata. Partly this is just provocative exhibitionism, but there is also deliberate repudiation of her own culture. Its place is filled by anxious flitting between material excess and different sources of spiritual comfort, cults and mysteries, Christianity and Judaism, ashtanga yoga and her 'kabbalistic' practices.

'What I practise has to do with something deeper than religion,' Madonna has claimed – but from the outside it looks typical of the West's jumble-sale approach to the human spirit.

Madonna's adoptive children owe her their deliverance from enormous material exigency, and that cannot be undervalued. But whatever else they may have lacked, they did once have the chance to feel attached to a place, a people, a culture of their own. It is hard to argue that they have not been severed from this, much as we may hope they will flourish without it, or find their own way to reconnect.

In the West, the bonds of kinship, place and history are increasingly regarded as irrelevant, illusory, even responsible for centuries of xenophobic prejudice. Our new 'anywhere' society is purported to supersede all this: dislocation from your own people is a small price to pay to become an individual; the loss of your own culture will be richly compensated when you graduate as a citizen of the world.

An alternative view was offered by the philosopher Simone Weil. Dr Highbrow directed me to her 1949 work, *The Need for Roots*, because he felt it illuminated many of the differences between life in Malaŵi and Europe. Weil, a gifted classicist, was born to affluent French-Jewish parents in 1909. Her influences were many, and she embraced aspects of her Jewish heritage as well as Catholicism and Marxism, eastern religion, ancient literature and trade unionism. But she gave herself seriously to all of these, whether as a scholar of Greek and Sanskrit, as a writer of challenging philosophy, as an austere devotee of religion or as a labourer in a Renault factory, at which she worked herself to illness and an early death out of solidarity with the proletariat.

In *The Need for Roots*, Weil identifies and describes the various requirements of the soul, laying out a vision of human fulfilment that emphasises spiritual over physical nourishment. Her perception of these demands is not unique, but she delineates them clearly and thoughtfully, and in ways that can be frighteningly practical, for example in her emphasis on labour and death as mankind's two paths to atonement.

So much in Weil's vision depends on the integrity of the community and its connectedness with the past. 'One sack of corn can always be substituted for another sack of corn', but the spiritual wealth inherited from the ancestors and stored as culture is irreplaceable: 'The future brings us nothing, gives us nothing; it is we who in order to build it have to give it everything, our very life. But to be able to give up, one has to possess; and we possess no other life, no other living sap, than the treasures stored up from the past and digested, assimilated and created afresh by us. Of all the human soul's needs, none is more vital than this one of the past.'

Uprootedness was, for Weil, the most dangerous malady that could afflict a society, because it was a self-propagating one. Whoever is uprooted, she observed, has a tendency, whether deliberate or not, to uproot others. And then you are left only with scattered individuals, colliding briefly and meaninglessly, like atoms in a void.

'I hate individualism,' declared the Malaŵian writer and intellectual Levi Mumba, another of Robert Laws' Livingstonia graduates. 'The European came with his individualism and thrust it on the native [. . .] It has suddenly torn the son from the father, or one man from another.' Mumba was writing in the 1920s, long before his country had to contend with the author of 'Bitch I'm

Madonna', 'Take a Bow', 'Material Girl' and 'Express Yourself'.

Madonna has been generous with her wealth, and that must always be borne in mind, but this book is about how we engage with other cultures. That engagement can be done well, in a manner mutually uplifting and beneficial, but it can also be done catastrophically, as Weil and Mumba warn. It is seldom a question of money; and some things, once broken, cannot be fixed with all the wealth in the world.

I thought of Sangala's people, of Lysard Moyo and his daughter, of Flemings and his adopted children, all united through shared experience, their own and that of generations past. They seemed so resilient, but how would they fare if their bonds to each other were ever dissolved? Then I thought of the Fax Machine to God, the irruption of a divisive cult with its strange imprecations to an alien deity. It might respond occasionally, even fleetingly appear, but would then always be conveyed back to the heavens by private jet. It was munificent to some degree, but jealous of other gods, and hungry for sacrifice.

XXVI

PALACES IN THE JUNGLE

'Here. This little pocket's been discreetly tucked away next to the crotch. It's specially designed to hold a single condom. All this underwear is from a hundred per cent fair-trade fabric, and it's all endorsed by Britney Starlet – yes, it's got the Britney Starlet underwear range label. She's been a big supporter of the whole project, especially the birth-control stuff. Britney is a *massive* advocate for women's rights back in the US, as I'm sure you know.'

We were on a tour of a village regeneration project sponsored by a small NGO; our young American guide, Mason, was the local director. He had been touting for visitors at a high-end safari lodge where we had been camping. His project was located just outside the gates of the park, and a 'village experience' was advertised at the lodge's reception alongside the elephant drives, bird walks, sundowners and more conventional safari activities. This was convenient for maximising visitors to the project, but also convenient for Mason, whose organisation paid for him to occupy one of the lodge's elegant chalets for the year he was working there. Normally you had to make a twenty-dollar donation to get the tour, but an unattached girl was travelling with our group and Mason had befriended her at the bar. As he wasn't busy that day, he waived the regular fee and said we should just donate what we felt like at the end of the afternoon.

The village itself was resplendent: roofs of brand-new corrugated aluminium glistened in the sun; the bricks were bright red and clearly not locally fired. The smart little houses had glass in the windows, drawn curtains, and robust doors that could be securely locked. To one side, an immense water butt stood on piers of steel and concrete, and was filled by an electric pump – 'when the power's actually running', Mason chuckled. All around were tiny plots of land, carefully marked out, blooming with a variety of produce.

'The great thing is that Britney got all her friends in Hollywood to subscribe to the project. So each of the plots you see has been individually sponsored by a different celebrity. There are some big names involved – you can read them all on the plaques over there.'

But their main contribution was prestige and moral support. The bulk of the funding came from a real-estate tycoon in the American Midwest. As Mason explained, she had visited Malaŵi several years before and been 'really upset by everything she saw'; she felt she had to do something to help. The result was an ersatz demonstration of what could be achieved if a single Malaŵian settlement was supported by virtually limitless overseas endowment.

We were shown photograph displays of the NGO's good works: the familiar shabby huts of mud and thatch which had existed before; the mighty lorries that had hauled over the expensive imported building materials; diggers going to work; smiling suntanned young Westerners constructing pit latrines on their gap years.

We were standing in the village 'community centre', but nobody else was there. Nor were they outside. The usual throng and bustle of the Malaŵian village were distinctly absent. The houses were clearly occupied, but were spaced far apart from each other by usual village standards, and were perhaps so commodious that their owners preferred to stay inside. Where I would have expected to see people gathered under the shade of trees, on their verandas, or in a communal arena, I saw just a couple of solitary, wandering youths. Mason called to one of them but was not heard immediately on account of a pair of oversized noise-cancelling headphones.

'Hey, chief! Jeffrey, right? What you doing?' Mason asked once the headphones were off.

Jeffrey murmured something inaudible.

'Nothing? Just chilling, right?'

'Ya!' he grinned.

'Where did you get those?' I asked, pointing to the headphones, which close-up looked in advanced disrepair.

'Britney Starlet!'

'And what are you listening to?'

Jeffrey smiled sheepishly and then laughed. He pulled the cable out of his trousers to show it was not attached to anything, just tucked in at the back. And then he went off, headphones back on, bobbing his head and beat-boxing to an imaginary accompaniment.

Malaŵi is a popular base for many foreign aid organisations. Bars and lodges are awash with Western aid workers, and the badges and slogans of their various organisations are omnipresent on the high-spec white 4x4s that sometimes outnumber all other vehicles on the road: the US Peace Corps, MSF, World Aid, World Vision, Raising Malaŵi, Build On – not to mention a plethora of smaller projects, some of which, like Mason's, might owe their existence to the wealth of just one individual. Since the fall of Banda, Malaŵi has become an established focus for these organisations because it is afflicted by all the problems they seek to alleviate while simultaneously offering a safe and stable environment in which to work. Life for Westerners in Malaŵi – as I discovered for myself – can also be very congenial. The country is warm, beautiful, relaxed. There are white sand beaches and elegant lakeshore lodges. In the big cities, you can find a bustling expatriate scene.

'They come here to do good,' commented Dr Highbrow, 'and they end up doing really rather well.'

Even besides recent egregious scandals at Oxfam, foreign aid organisations have for years become accustomed to adverse criticism. Their work is varied and sometimes very worthy, so why do they all get tarred with the same brush? The problem is cultural. First, there is a recurrence of the same ideological preoccupations, which obviously owe more to a Western agenda than to any local concerns: social justice, female empowerment, birth control, wealth inequality, battling homophobic prejudice. This gives to the whole of foreign intervention a monolithic character, even when individual organisations may be doing something different.

And then there is a homogeneity to the people employed in this industry. Excepting technically qualified workers like doctors and engineers, it is no caricature to observe that most aid workers are young, Western-educated to university level, usually in arts subjects or social sciences, with or without some postgraduate qualification in development studies. Coming from affluent, middle-class backgrounds, their outlooks and sensibilities are invariably 'progressive'. They are all overseas to correct the things they perceive to be wrong with the world, but their culture is supremely globalised, and, in Malaŵi, it collides with one that is quintessentially local.

Most of these expatriates stay in their host countries only fleetingly – three years is considered a long commitment to one place. Either they are doing a stint abroad before returning to 'real life' back at home, or they are dedicated aid industry professionals, in which case they move on and up the humanitarian career ladder, swapping one dysfunctional country for another every couple of years. 'Dystopophilia' was Dr Highbrow's name for it and, to a certain sort of person, it is a very appealing life. In fact, it was the sort of career I once imagined for myself before I chanced upon the advert for a job at Kamuzu Academy.

The transience of most aid workers' presence is a big problem in a society where so much is governed by personal contact. Within a tiny radius of my home, examples abounded of projects that had disintegrated because their sponsors oversaw them for so little time. When they left, there was usually a gap, and then a successor would begin the work of reinventing the wheel. In the meantime, tree plantations withered because they were left unwatered; libraries were turned into storage rooms; dairy goats were slaughtered for meat, solar panels sold off and beehives burnt for firewood.

Such short stays seldom result in mastery of any local language. Mine was no exception, and I found myself working hard to pretend it did not matter. After all, English is the country's official first language. But it is not widely spoken in the village, and almost all engagement between aid organisations and the rural population is mediated through bilingual locals. A Dutch friend, fresh out of university, ended up supervising a women's microfinance project for a year and described to me how it worked.

She was in charge of the pot of money, but, speaking no local language, she had to delegate all decisions about who should receive a loan to a self-appointed committee of older women, two of whom spoke fair English and claimed authority in the village. Trying to convene all the elders in one place took weeks of planning and negotiation, and this was the greatest demand on her time and energy. When finally assembled, the women would engage in protracted deliberation, the details of which were entirely opaque to my friend. Finally, they would summon her to communicate their decisions. The lucky young women selected to be beneficiaries would then form a queue to collect the tiny sums from the microfinance office. As she doled out the cash, my friend was offered only the vaguest explanation of how the money would be used, but all the recipients had learnt to deploy the talismanic word 'business' when they reached her desk. Later that day, one of the young women showed off what she had just bought. 'Look. I am carrying my *business* on my head,' she stated firmly. It was a bundle of groceries – her weekly shop.

Scarcely any of the 'loans' were ever repaid. But the impact was at least not as pernicious as at another microfinance project where a colleague of hers was working. There, it finally emerged, the old women were collating the funds to cover the overheads of a brothel they had been able to set up.

The unstated premise of the microfinance initiative was also subtly ideological: the women were supposed to possess greater financial acumen which, once liberated, would turn insignificant sums of money into thriving enterprise. All that was stopping them was the domination of their feckless menfolk. With this overcome, prosperity must ensue.

Such wishful thinking vitiated many projects. At a friend's hospital, a campaign to reduce maternal mortality offered a tiny cash bonus to mothers who came to have their children at the maternity unit rather than deliver at home. In so doing, they undermined a separate scheme to promote birth control. And down the road from where I lived, an infant nutrition project offered food vouchers to mothers whenever their children fell below a certain centile of weight to height ratio – with inevitable, tragic results.

When Western agendas are so pervasive, it becomes harder and harder to discriminate genuine local concerns, as their expression is distorted by alien needs and expectations. Malaŵians have quickly learnt, for example, that the largesse of passing foreigners is bestowed far more generously if you affirm that your efforts are directed towards the advancement of some fashionable cause. At a village in the south, I noted a sign for a 'Gender Sensitive Community Based Disaster Preparedness and Food Security Project', which had been endorsed by the EU's overseas development fund.

If local concerns ever are identified, it sometimes feels as if they are actively disdained. Malaŵi is a socially conservative country that places great value on propriety and courtesy. Mason's condom underwear was offensive and patronising, with its coy insinuation that Malaŵians were so governed by animal appetites that they would only think of contraception if it was physically present in their underpants. There was once a similarly insensitive poster campaign in South Africa, which promoted birth control with the slogan: 'Africa Needs More Oral Sex'.

The reflex among many young foreigners in Malaŵi is that local values stand in need of correction and that their own role in the country is to challenge them, in preparation for replacement with those of the West. The last British High Commissioner was a young woman who caused widespread offence when, soon after her appointment, she tweeted her disgust at a traditional form of greeting demonstrated by a Tonga woman who was meeting the country's vice president. The greeting, photographs of which appeared in national newspapers, involved the woman abasing herself in the dust before the minister's feet. It was an image that might make many Westerners uncomfortable. But Malaŵians were angered by the newcomer's self-righteous aspersions, and they retaliated on social media, pointing out her arrogance and ignorance. From a newly appointed diplomat, the incident was not suggestive of sympathy with the local culture, which Malaŵians naturally took her to despise.

'One must not be afraid of anything that is really there,' wrote William Johnson. 'Good and bad must be united in our comprehension [. . .] One must not try to get rid of the people while one delights in the beauty of their hills.'

Too few modern visitors to Malaŵi have inherited the tolerance enjoined by Johnson. Their concerns and attitudes are imported from home and seldom re-examined in the light of new surroundings. Sometimes this can have hilarious results, as when a young English aid worker, who briefly lived near me, gave an impromptu lecture on human rights law to her village elders. It was on the day when news emerged of the death of Osama bin Laden, and the head master of the local school unwisely tried to congratulate her on that great victory for her country. 'Mr Madimba!' she huffed in outrage. 'Are you seriously telling me that you see nothing wrong with state-sponsored assassination?'

Malaŵi is widely considered to be in a condition of perpetual demographic crisis, with overpopulation placing a massive strain on land supply, healthcare and the environment. The case for birth control may well be irresistible. But all too often, well-intentioned projects betray a lack of deep reflection on the societies they seek to engineer. Near where I lived, a shiny NGO sign advertised vasectomy with the furtively reproachful slogan: 'For men who love their wives!'

The bonds that hold people together are complex, even mysterious. They have evolved over generations, like the interlinked components of a delicate ecosystem. Would anyone, least of all a passing foreigner, notice their dissolution? Sangala's *gule* party was a violent celebration of fecundity, to which men and women, young and old gave themselves unreservedly. It amplified the fortitude and vitality of that small, long-suffering community. Similarly for Flemings and Lysard Moyo, a superabundance of children might have been the ultimate good in their lives. Campaigns for birth control meddle with such deep existential reflexes as these. But a certain type of young aid worker enjoins Africans to give up their own notions of fulfilment, so that he can return to Europe in triumph to report an improved infant mortality statistic. By way of compensation, he leaves behind only the lingering odour of his own culture, with its promise of material satisfactions which, for most Malaŵians, remain unattainable.

Interventionist arguments may well outweigh these considerations. But aid organisations could certainly act with greater caution and humility, with an awareness that things might be more complicated than are dreamt of in their philosophy and a readiness to be around to pick up the pieces when things go wrong.

There were of course no more momentous interventions than the elimination of slavery and the Christianisation of Africa. These were also driven by an alien agenda; and there are some, within the discipline of post-colonial studies, who dispute whether they were ultimately for good or ill. Whatever the final judgement, it was done in a different spirit and by a different sort of person. And what men like Laws, Scott and Maples *did* get right might be instructive for us today.

Johnson's sternest warning to his fellow missionaries was to 'fear ourselves' – a cultural principle of 'first do no harm'. This did not mean he deprecated the technical and educational superiority he brought with him. But his and Laws' journals abound with equivocation and self-doubt about the tasks they were engaged in, even after many decades. Despite this, they worked tirelessly, embraced hardship, even gave their lives – it was part of the job. It is hard to have faith in proselytisers who come and go, enjoying privilege and amusement, sacrificing nothing.

They might deprecate 'voluntourism', but foreign aid workers often look like they're on holiday, and the worldliness they claim is closely related to the number of exotic destinations they have managed to visit. Being 'well travelled' is for them a *sine qua non*, yet the places they stay and the sorts of people they meet across the world are almost indistinguishable – as I knew well from my own travels.

The 'backpacker lodges' where they gather, sometimes even live, are all alike, from Tanzania to Thailand, from Bali to Brazil. In Malaŵi, they are clustered around places on the lake first settled by hippies drifting through in the 1970s. Today there is still a pose of anti-materialist spirit, but the lodge-owners also seek profit, and the premium they charge is for provision of the familiar. The owners and visitors must be Westerners who are young in age, or at least in spirit. Locals are essential for colour, but white people must make up a critical mass: it is to be their safe space – a haven amid Third World dysfunctionality. There is always the same distinct iconography: wood is prominent, with its suggestion of ecological friendliness, signs are painted in a sloppy yellow, red and green script to evoke a relaxed Caribbean vibe, and the food must be excellent, with vegan options and cold beer. Wi-Fi is hopefully available, and there might be meaningless slogans behind the bar about the power of love. If the lodge gets the formula right, its custom will snowball as like attracts like. Occasionally Malaŵian proprietors try to get in on the act, but they seldom achieve the same success.

An English aid worker, grizzled and dread-locked, is communicating local knowledge to a pretty Canadian girl, smiling and jejune. A tanned Euro couple lie self-absorbed and resplendent on the sand. Some Asian Americans are getting advice from a worldly Australian, who has a Burmese mantra tattooed on one arm and a Norse fertility symbol on the other. Their conversations are unvarying: gossip about holiday romances and fussing over Skype connections; a Spanish girl enthuses about yoga, a Dane about capoeira; Americans apologise to anyone who will listen for the existence of Donald Trump. It is a cocoon of jolly volunteer projects interspersed with parties, beach ball, drinking games, cliff dives, giant Jenga – all played out to the unrelenting rhythms of Bob Marley.

The fantasy is of rich and vibrant diversity; in reality, these lodges are at least as parochial and exclusive as the clubs set up by British colonialists throughout the Empire. In most cases, the only possible cultural engagement comes through a carefully regulated number of 'beach boys' who are granted admission to supply drugs and some local frisson. These are 'Palaces in the Jungle', observed Felix Mnthali:

> [. . .] and here are the revellers
> who have foregathered
> to wine and dine
> on our sweat; they dance
> and make merry sometimes
> strip for orgies
> on our sweat and blood
> No, no don't call it tomfoolery
> call it "technical assistance"

> or partnership in progress
> for how else can Africa go forward
> [. . .]
> From now on
> we shall wake up wondering
> [. . .]
> where all that money went
> and they will wake up wondering
> what paradise is reserved
> for those who come to help.

Sugar-and-Spice got his name from a stoned English expatriate who bought his weed when he was just starting off in the business. They smoked together on the beach and laughed hysterically as his customer rechristened him in allusion to the 'all things nice' which he purveyed. It is a joke he has since reprised with every customer he has had. The Englishman was based in the capital and revisited the lake many times. When his stint in Malaŵi came to an end, he left Sugar-and-Spice an email address and never replied to any of his messages.

Sugar-and-Spice now just loafs around the backpacker lodge. His lank clothing and shifty bloodshot eyes bring an insalubrious character to the place, but he also sells weed to the owner so is one of the few Africans permitted past the sign at the gate which reads: 'Right of Entry Reserved'.

The Euro couple ignore him. An English party, nursing hangovers, groan their dismissal but vaguely indicate they might look him up later. Some girls briefly flirt and then grow irritated because he lingers. Then an NGO worker greets him as a long-lost friend before bargaining for his wares.

Marijuana is harshly censured in Malaŵian society as a road to perdition. Its use is uncommon, except in areas where Westerners are concentrated – and there it is used and trafficked widely. It might seem easy money, but the life of European dissipation is addictive and debilitating, and the beach boys often look washed out by middle age, if they even live that long. I sometimes came across them in hospitals, and a single item of clothing in the Rastafarian colours of red, yellow and green would all too often betoken drink and drug problems, or HIV. On occasion, they were accompanied by relatives: Yes, he had been smoking *chamba* for several years. No, he was fine before that.

Weed is just part of a broader Western lifestyle in which Africans are essential for cosmesis, but can never properly participate. Cultural nomadism depends on freedom of movement and a bank account in the West; only then can you afford to dabble in a chilled-out life abroad, confident in the security you will return to when the party is over. For most Malaŵians, an airline ticket is completely unaffordable, let alone what would be required to qualify for a visa. And so they dabble in the holiday lifestyle tantalisingly exhibited before them. But when the foreigners depart, the locals discover that the hedonism is fleeting and the fraternity illusory. They are left with only the hollow, dementing jingle that never leaves the airwaves: 'Don't worry 'bout a thing! 'Cos every little thing gonna be alright!'

XXVII

IMPERIAL FOLLY

Malaŵi was absorbed into the British Empire in 1891, at the height of the infamous 'Scramble for Africa'. Yet it was with some reluctance that Lord Salisbury's government assumed control: there were no glittering resources, as in South Africa, nor was it a land for settlers, like Kenya or Rhodesia. Malaŵi became a 'protectorate' – a term which can arouse skepticism, but needs to be understood in context.

Missionaries and their supporters came to desire an official British presence in order to maintain peace in the region, eliminate slavery and pre-empt the expansionism of others. Besides the centuries-old Arab slave trade, for several decades the peoples of Malaŵi had also been predated upon by tribes of the Zulu diaspora, migrating from the south. From Mozambique, the Portuguese were extending the frontiers of their possessions, everywhere imposing forced labour and a cruel penal code that drove many to flee in search of better conditions under British rule. To the north, the Germans had carved out a vast territory – modern-day Tanzania – where they ruled with brutality and routinely faced widespread insurrection. By contrast, Malaŵi saw only a little violence, and it was mostly directed at slavers.

White landowners were few and concentrated in pockets, mostly in the south. There were no incentives to promote immigration; on the contrary, a colonial office prospectus from the 1900s gloomily urged would-be settlers to think twice about coming at all. The land was undeveloped, it pointed out; disease was rampant, life was tough, and large amounts of private capital would be needed to start any enterprise at all. Gold-diggers, good-timers and speculators were warned of disappointment.

Nevertheless, a colonial society did emerge, its rule underpinned by exploitation and racial injustice, as elsewhere. The wisest missionaries often equivocated about their own presence in the country, but for colonists and administrators, whether well intentioned or not, there was little doubt about their right to rule and profit.

Cecil Rhodes maintained a watchful eye, in case any valuable minerals were found, but it soon became clear that the country's major commodity was its workforce. Shortages of labour, rather than of land, were then the major limitation on most colonial economies in the region. In Malaŵi, young men were relatively numerous and, soon, unusually well educated, thanks to missionary endeavours like that at Livingstonia. They were enabled and encouraged to leave the country and seek employment in South Africa and the Rhodesias, where they became farm and factory managers, railway and mining clerks – like Kamuzu Banda. They were often much better paid than the local people they took charge of, so when Banda got his scholarship to America, some of his peers were astonished that he wanted to give up a good and steady salary in Johannesburg for the uncertainties and challenges of life elsewhere.

But while its skilled labour fed the prosperity of nearby British colonies, Malaŵi itself went undeveloped by the colonial government. The country was bled of its ablest young men, and when they did return home, a measure of social upheaval was inevitable. The predominant Chewa people had practised a system of uxorilocality, in which a wife's blood relations could make a strong claim on the husband's assets. But this arrangement began to break down when the men came back from abroad, seeking wives but now determined to guard their new wealth jealously. They had become rich by local standards, in part by learning the ways of others – hence the lament of Levi Mumba about the intrusion of 'European individualism' into traditional life.

Perhaps the greatest injustice of colonial rule in Malaŵi was land seizure, seldom achieved by force but often by trickery, sometimes on a massive scale – though even at its peak, only a small proportion of the country was in the hands of settlers. Nevertheless, the missionaries gave white incomers a reputation for probity, and many took ruthless advantage of this, inviting chiefs to make their marks on ruinous contracts in exchange for beads and calico. At a place called Magomero, relatives of David Livingstone claimed over 160,000 acres for themselves.

Once the estates were founded, the tenants – many of whom were economic migrants – found themselves vulnerable to exploitation. Their landlords claimed rent, which they expected to be paid in labour. As the years went by, the demands on their time increased, and their own smallholdings were neglected in proportion as they toiled for the profit of white men. Defaulters might be evicted from their homes, and troublemakers flogged.

This system of labour – known as *thangata* – was eventually prohibited by the colonial government but, while it lasted, made a mockery of the elevated principles which had inspired British involvement in the country at the beginning. As David Clement Scott observed, it was 'the yoke of a new slaver'.

The local conception of land ownership was communal,

he pointed out, and European property laws were based on incomprehensibly foreign principles. Few understood what they were letting themselves in for when they signed their names to agreements with white land-grabbers. The iniquity was obvious, Scott went on, and indeed it was 'to the native's credit that he did not understand what lay beneath the documents to which he affixed his mark'.

Scott tried to insist that settlers uphold the same moral standard as the missionaries who had paved their entry to the country. 'Immorality should be ground for dismissal,' he urged, 'otherwise we shall come to social and commercial wreck upon the irrefragable rock of God's commandment!'

As we have seen, it was Scott who was 'wrecked' when the white settlers identified him as a thorn in their side and conspired to drive him out. But by then he had already infected Malaŵian apprentices with his high-mindedness; they would soon become the instruments of national independence and the vindicators of his sense of justice.

But even idealists like Scott and Johnson recognised that commerce was necessary to make their moral endeavours viable. Unlike today's foreign aid workers, they did not envisage their work being sustained indefinitely by other people's money. And they noted that slavery recrudesced wherever the British presence faltered or withdrew. The settlers brought the greed and ugliness of capitalism but also its benefits: development, technical advance and the security fostered when interests become vested.

As usual, the benefits of capitalism were experienced in unequal measure – an inequality which was more flagrant because apportioned along lines of colour. Yet nobody emerged grotesquely rich from Malaŵi, as Rhodes did from South Africa, not to mention Leopold from the Congo. Most ventures struggled or failed, and the colony was overall run at a loss to the British exchequer. For this reason, settlers remained few. Besides missionaries, most Europeans in Malaŵi were administrators.

These young men had signed up for a life with the colonial service, stereotypically after studying Classics at Oxbridge. They were assigned a spot on the globe and – after some brief training – sent to look after it. A Colonial Office guide from 1922 for new appointees to Malaŵi tried to give a sense of their duties: repairing roads and bridges lost to flood, holding inquests, investigating claims to chieftainship, inspecting prisons, supervising local council elections, mediating between white landowners and their workers, providing emergency care following a bus crash, building a reservoir or tracking down a lost suitcase – all to be performed by a young Englishman in his early twenties working on his own in the bush.

We shudder today to imagine entire nations being governed in this way, and the impact – especially psychological – has been well described. Yet the system worked, after a fashion, and it was not wholly ill-intentioned. The Colonial Office made clear early on that its role was to pave the way for self-government. In the same prospectus for new appointees, it was noted that there had already emerged among Malaŵians 'the development of political consciousness and the clamour for realisation of their new desires'. These were 'fully susceptible of guidance in the best interests of the country and its people', and it was 'the prime duty of the administrative officer to recognise such thoughts and movements, understand their origins, and to guide them with sympathy and foresight'.

Command of local languages was essential, and officials had to pass a series of increasingly challenging exams in the first few years of their service. Perhaps more importantly, they had to possess and cultivate certain personal qualities which were also identified in the Colonial Office prospectus:

'patience, tolerance, humour, integrity, tenacity of purpose – the administrative officer must be, quite simply, a good man'. Such down-to-earth requirements as these seldom feature in job adverts issued by today's foreign NGOs in Africa, which might speak instead of the need to be 'passionate' about the work of international development. Yet how few of their employees devote their entire lives to public service far from home in the manner of these peculiar, far-flung Britons.

But against their daily bread of derring-do, you often detect something humdrum about these young men. The old colonial capital was Zomba, a cool and elegant town, picturesquely nestled low on the slopes of an immense plateau which lours above, beset by mists and pine trees. At the old gymkhana club, you can see where the colonial elite once congregated on breaks from their districts to immerse themselves in English triviality: among dark wood panelling and billiard tables, beneath hunting prints and the gaze of the King Emperor's portrait, they chattered ceaselessly about cricket elevens and rugby fifteens, affairs and grudges, servant problems and tennis-court maintenance – the boorishness fired by endless rounds of whisky stengahs, bitters and gin.

You get the impression of a small insular community whose lifeblood was curtain-twitching and petty rivalry in dinner invitations and golf-course precedence. The town was so arranged that the sprawling mass of native dwellings lay at the bottom of the hill. Above them was an Indian quarter, occupying much of the town proper and bustling with shophouses, markets and mosques. Above this, the houses of British officials were arranged on the slopes of the plateau, each with a tidy lawned garden and sweeping views over the plains. They were allocated according to rank, from the governor's castellated pile at the top to the humble bungalows of new arrivals at the bottom. Every death, promotion, resignation and retirement was occasion for excited speculation at the possibility of being shuffled to a more coveted position higher up the hill. The town has a reassuring atmosphere of order and reliability but betrays an obsession with hierarchy that borders on the neurotic.

Yet there were settlers and officials who rose above the fug of booze and gossip to engage more thoughtfully with the culture around them. Sir Harry Johnston is an ambiguous figure, but perhaps the first Englishman to approach Malaŵi with the sustained curiosity of the ethnographer. His background was humble; his self-advancement began when he won a place at Stockwell Grammar School in South London, after which he went on to study fine art at the Royal Academy. He also had an intrepid character, delighted in foreign languages and hankered after the exotic. Adventure took him to Malaŵi, where he played a picaresque part in the wars against the slavers and became the country's first governor. At the same time he was also recording everything he saw, from bird life to tribal markings, the fighting gear of warriors and the adornments of their women, the rituals of chieftainship and the lurid punishments of the slavers. His writing has a lyrical quality that often veers into sensationalism, but his wonder and delight have the ring of sincerity.

It was the last generation of British settlers and officials, however, who really devoted themselves to celebration of the local culture. Perhaps they were aware of the sunset of European supremacy so could approach Malaŵi in a humbler, more receptive way. Their contributions trickled in from all over the country to fill the pages of the *Nyasaland* (later, *Society of Malawi*) *Journal* – a wondrous compendium of patient observation and research that endures to this day. All knew the country and its languages well; each also devoted himself to expertise in some tiny area of Malaŵian life, whether history, prehistory, butterflies, birds, inheritance law, ethno-musicology, geomorphology, or dance.

W.H.J. Rangeley was District Commissioner at Nkhotakhota in the period just before independence. Born in Zambia but educated at Oxford, he had a foot in both worlds and applied himself to the study of Chewa culture with both and enthusiasm and academic rigor. His was the first substantial effort to understand and describe *gule wamkulu*, and Dr Highbrow was delighted to discover that the secret language of the Nyau, which Rangeley deciphered, was still current when he conducted research of his own in the area around Kamuzu Academy.

Rangeley's interest in *gule* was deep but retained the propriety and distance of the level-headed colonial official. Unlike that contemporary scholar of *gule*, Claude Boucher at Mua, he never sought initiation into Nyau. But another Englishman lacked Rangeley's restraint, and found himself tragically out of his depth in the local culture. In the national archives at Kew, I found a slim file concerning what is referred to as 'the unfortunate case of Mr Racey'.

Racey was a young official sent to Chikwawa, then a deeply inhospitable corner of southern Malaŵi, being hot, humid, malarial and cut off from the rest of the country by a tall, steep escarpment. It is also renowned, even today, for the activity of its witches and the potency of its magic. A friend of mine has himself witnessed there the administration of *mwabvi* – the poisonous bark used for trial by ordeal to identify a witch.

Within Racey's district was a shrine devoted to the worship of M'bona, a hero of ancient legend, who had been decapitated in time of drought but whose blood then gushed forth to replenish lakes and rivers, restoring plenty to the land. M'bona's martyrdom became an important component of local religion, celebrated at several shrines in central and southern Malaŵi. Worship was directed by virginal rain priestesses, wedded to the spirit of M'bona, and connected to each other across the ages through metempsychosis. The cult may or may not be extant today. Boucher photographed some shrines during the 1980s – shambolic little houses of mud, stick and grass, just two feet high, and located in tiny forest clearings. But the humbleness of the dwellings was deceptive: the spirit power contained therein was purported to be very strong indeed.

The file contains Racey's journal from 1904, apparently intended as notes for a study of the cult. He begins to visit the shrine, at first in a spirit of dispassionate enquiry. He notes the initial reluctance of his guides to take him there, and the reticence of the priestess when addressed. Eventually he acquires the etiquette required to approach her, learns to adorn himself sombrely, to make condign offerings, and discovers details of the cult's operation. He describes its reputed powers to do good or harm, bring rain or ruin, direct witches, man and beasts. All is described lucidly at first, in a tidy, copperplate script.

Then, over the course of several visits, Racey begins to notice odd occurrences. He traces these back to an occasion when, walking through the forest to reach the shrine, he was struck suddenly by a painful headache, which he describes as like something trying to bore itself into his head. The headache passes and he resumes his visit, which is otherwise uneventful. On another occasion, walking in the same forest, he finds a decapitated snake lying in his path.

The script from then on betrays a growing unease that develops into wild agitation. The ink is more and more often smudged, the letters become disordered, the page sometimes indented with the force of the nib, as Racey describes still stranger happenings. A hideous beast darts across his path and then leaps with impossible acrobatic skill up a rock face at the edge of the forest. At first he gets only a glimpse as it passes in a flash. When he sees it again, it has 'short white glossy hair, the head of a sea horse, eyes horrid red, legs and feet of a lion, small wings, and long white tail with nippers and stings on the end'.

It becomes clear that Racey is suffering a complete psychotic breakdown. His experiences become hallucinatory, his beliefs delusional, his writings so deranged as to constitute a textbook case of formal thought disorder.

At times he is aware of his madness and wrestles against it. There is a suggestion that he seeks help from a local medicine man, obtaining a preparation of bark and herbs to cure him of his possession. At other times he seems to attempt a plaintive reconciliation with his own religion, insisting: 'I must continue to write as a child of the Almighty, otherwise what there is to be said will not be clear!'

There are periodic struggles to recover the outlook of the ethnographer with which he started. But the trajectory is all towards insanity. He discovers a power to produce 'a few drops of rain'; and starts to see 'crawling and shuffling things', which try to ensnare him in his hammock or with his butterfly and mosquito nets. The last entry in the journal, written at the peak of the hot season, notes some local claims about the spirits of dead people wandering in the village. 'I have not seen this!' he insists, but then immediately contradicts himself, admitting that he did see the spirit of a recently deceased friend of his – 'and it was covered with snakes and horrible creatures'. These are the last words of the journal.

The next item in the file is correspondence between the colony's chief medical officer and various government officials, and a note that records Racey's repatriation to England and referral to a London specialist.

The cause of Racey's madness is impossible to determine. Perhaps he brought a predisposition to mental illness with him when he went to Africa. What rings clear through his demented writings is his terrible isolation in a remote and bewildering world. And there is a particular pathos: while he was losing his mind in Chikwawa, other colleagues of his were probably drinking and boasting in the gymkhana club in the capital, blithely incurious about the strangeness around them. Racey did try to connect, but he lacked the anchorage in his own world from which to venture out and explore another with safety.

XXVIII

CORNSTALK & LEAF

White farmers had all but vanished from Malaŵi when I lived there. There had never been more than a few hundred, and these seldom prospered as elsewhere on the continent. 'It has become clearer every year that Nyasaland is not a country for the small European settler,' noted the Colonial Office in the 1930s. 'European agriculture except for tea is virtually an economic failure.' Even in its least profitable forms, the idea of white farming in Africa makes us uncomfortable today. The odour of racial injustice and exploitation is not easily dissipated. But farming demands a commitment to the land and some achievement of harmony with others who dwell on it, and I was curious to know how this had been done by complete outsiders in an unfamiliar world. Through Dr Highbrow, I became acquainted with Tom and Flora Pastime, perhaps the last of their breed in the whole country.

To buy a pack of butter sometimes felt like a tiny feat of heroism. The favourable outcome of this mission, which for me involved a journey of almost 150 miles, depended on the smile of fortune through numberless vicissitudes. At any point you could be thwarted by conditions of road and weather, the failure of your vehicle, unavailability of fuel at the depot or of paper money at the bank, of the supply of electricity and, naturally, of butter. I once got to the end of my journey to find there had been an extended power cut in the capital: the butter had all spoiled in the tropical heat for want of refrigeration. Worse still, the phone network was down, and I could get no fuel for the return journey because the pumps could not run. As I was living in Malaŵi for a few years only, I almost relished this as part of the rich carnival of daily life. But the whole rigmarole seemed a bit silly after I first visited the Pastimes' estate in the Shire Highlands.

They did not depend on the vagaries of a dysfunctional supermarket in a distant city. Knowing they would spend their whole lives in Malaŵi, they had found it more expedient to clear land, lay pasture, build dairy sheds, import cattle, train milkmaids and start churning. When we first met, there were buttered finger sandwiches and scones with mulberry jam and clotted cream for tea.

They were in their late eighties. Flora had been born in Malaŵi to an English farming family, and Tom had met her there when he went out after the war as a policeman. A few years later, they had bought their own land to farm for themselves. Their estate was large by the standards of England, small by those of Africa.

From the tarmac main road, you could see nothing of their house, even though the landscape all around had been denuded for firewood, as elsewhere in Malaŵi. Some way down the long laterite drive, you crossed the brow of a small hill and were suddenly plunged into gentle woods and rolling fields that might have been in southern England. Jerseys and Herefords rejoiced in succulent grass, glowing green in the brilliant sun. Adjacent fields were dense with tobacco, beyond which lay tall thickets of blue gums. The road took you up to a hillock, peppered with the red cherries of coffee bushes nestled in the shade of banana palms. At the top was the house, a sprawling bungalow of weathered brick, with a wide veranda stretching round all sides. A pair of thoroughbred horses nuzzled each other in a paddock right at the front.

Inside, a vast fireplace was flanked by two mighty elephant tusks, a roaring lion's head above. Suspended beside them were 'olde English' hunting prints and horse brasses. Tom sat in a large armchair hung with a bright starched antimacassar; behind him spears and knobkerries were arranged among twee portraits of family dogs and horses. An elderly major-domo answered a service bell and brought tea.

For several years before and after independence, Tom had worked for the outgoing British administration, and then for Dr Banda. We sat beside the crackling fire as he recalled how he was once present at a dinner hosted for the new leader by the outgoing British governor, Sir Glyn Jones, who had spent almost his entire life in Africa. There had been a playful exchange in which Banda, who had just returned home after his absence of forty years in the West, laboriously explained the meaning of a Malaŵian proverb. Jones, who knew it well, listened patiently and then teasingly countered with an explanation of an English proverb. Banda smiled politely before retaliating in kind, and so it went on. Tom reckoned that the two men (who were becoming close friends) were both delighting in the irony that Banda knew Britain better than the governor and that the governor knew Malaŵi better than Banda.

Tom had been a policeman but also served for a time as Banda's personal pilot. He had then busied himself with the construction of tiny airfields in far-flung corners of the country. For the last forty years, though, he and his wife had devoted themselves to farming and were still hard at work. I was woken at five the next day by a gentle knock on my door. I opened it to find a pot of tea laid on a trestle outside.

Half an hour later, the house was busy with activity, and we were soon setting out on a tour of the farm.

Flora had been crippled by childhood polio and had walked with a stick ever since. Now she was further assisted by a Great Dane, who cleaved to her side, keeping his head rigid and upright so she could lean on it for stability. So supported, she shambled between pigsty, cowshed and hen coop while Tom busied himself with the nurseries and tobacco sheds. There were over a hundred Malaŵians living on the estate, including children and wives of the tenant farmers, and everyone greeted her affectionately as she limped by. Both she and Tom spoke two local languages fluently, though with clipped English accents. In fact, everyone I met on the estate was at least bilingual.

After four hours, we reconvened for a gargantuan meal of porridge, eggs, bacon, sausages, fruit and jam, washed down with gallons of coffee. Only the HP Sauce came from the outside world. After breakfast, work was resumed, and I joined Tom on his round with one of the farm managers, a softly spoken Malaŵian of about forty called Frederick. He and his wife had both been born on a neighbouring estate, now vanished – dissolved into scrub and smallholdings. As a young man, Frederick had travelled to Zambia and worked on a vast commercial farm there. When, after a few years, he had wanted to return to Malaŵi, he was welcomed by the Pastimes, and was now well established on their land with a large family. He showed me his cottage: a robust, elegant bungalow typical of those built in the colonial period, with whitewashed walls and sage green roof and windows. He offered his apologies: his wife had left early with the milk float into town, but he introduced several of his children, who were playing and tinkering in their abundant kitchen garden. His oldest daughter, he was proud to explain, had recently left to study in South Africa.

We walked on, with Tom and Frederick pointing out various important features of the estate. A dam of massive, rough stones formed a reservoir from which sprang a complex irrigation system of trickling streams. There were forests of pine for timber, and of blue gum, to feed the flues in four brick tobacco-curing factories, which teetered and smoked with a vaguely Dickensian character. Other fields had been left fallow, and there was much discussion of prospective yields, both men quoting obscure agronomic principles.

At the heart of the estate, several acres surrounding a swamp were kept undisturbed as a refuge for wildlife: the whole swathe of land, densely tangled with lianas and thorn-bushes, was all but impenetrable. It had become a refuge for leopards, and I was blithely advised to take a stout stick with me if strolling at dusk: 'If the leopard lunges, just hit it. On the nose.'

There were many thickets of trees, and the estate teemed and chattered with finches and wagtails, swallows and swifts. As we walked through a spinney of acacias, we startled a pair of hammerkops building their huge, elaborate nest. Tom was a keen ornithologist and could spot and identify tiny indistinct creatures at astonishing distances; however, his love of birds was also of the sort that had no qualms about killing them. He and Frederick spent a long time discussing the need for more cover around the lake to facilitate duck shoots.

Tom's greatest pride was his stables. He and Flora had both been riding until just the year before, when he had a fall and Flora had developed a leg ulcer. Still, there was no question of giving the horses up. Indeed one of his Lipizzaner mares had just given birth. A new stable boy was being trained, and, when we arrived, an elderly groom was supervising the young man in examining the foal's hooves. Tom's consolation for having stopped riding was now to teach it to any of the farm lads who wanted to work with horses. He showed me the field set up for dressage and indicated a small mound where he would sit on his shooting stick and instruct the pupil through an antique brass megaphone.

The days end early in Malaŵi. The sun begins to set before five, leaving less than an hour before complete darkness. We were back at the house in good time and found a retired bishop had come over for tea. Then the local police chief stopped by on his way home from work, and so we all sat on the veranda for a drink. It seemed a moment crystallised from the past: khaki and polished leather, clerical collar and purple shirt, the babble of the wireless, lime juice and gin. Did someone say something about the gold standard?

And then it was night. Before bed, there was an hour with the photograph album beside the guttering fire. A Brahms piano concerto thundered from a cassette player, and I noticed the complete works of Thomas Mann in German on the bookshelves. Tom had served in intelligence during the war, and the album contained unexpected snaps of post-war Austria and Italy. There were also innumerable photographs of dogs and horses, their lineages traced and argued about by the couple in obsessive detail. But it was the pictures of Malaŵi that interested me. There were images of the remote mountain plateaux where Tom had staked out and tested rough grass airstrips. In other photos, he appeared with Dr Banda, accompanied by police officers black and white, at ceremonies and tours of inspection. In one picture, the two men stand face to face, staring fixedly at each other as Tom salutes his new chief with a sword held rigidly upright between them.

'I felt I never got to know him. He was quiet. Aloof.

Enigmatic. But Mama and her uncle were always very friendly.'

Above all, though, the album contained images of the estate when Tom and his wife first bought it. It had been complete wilderness, as dense and forbidding as the preserved wildlife refuge I had been shown that afternoon. The vegetation was laboriously cleared, but the land was still strewn with boulders. 'That one was too big to move,' Tom commented on a photograph of a block of granite the size of a house. It filled the space now occupied by the reservoir. 'We had to dynamite it.' In the next photo, workers were refashioning the blasted fragments to form a mighty dry stone wall I remembered from the morning.

The order which the Pastimes had wrought from chaos was extraordinary, even miraculous to me. Their lives' work had been to achieve a state of bountiful autarky by which they supported themselves and a host of other families. But an enormous disparity was obvious, between tenants and masters, black and white. Indeed, the whole arrangement had a racialised, feudal character. But Tom and Flora's privilege was precarious: the financial viability of the farm had long hung in the balance, the profits of one year going to pay the debts accrued in the last. They could probably never sell the land, not that they wanted to. And the example of nearby countries suggested their right of ownership might easily become vulnerable. Their children had dispersed in pursuit of better prospects and security abroad.

As we sat chatting, I found myself contemplating the oozing bandages wrapped round Flora's suppurating leg, elevated on a foot-stool beside her sleeping dog. The couple were advancing into old age and infirmity but could avail themselves of little better healthcare than their tenants. I asked if they had thought of leaving at independence. 'Very briefly, I suppose,' Flora answered, 'but we never really wanted to.' What about after the fall of Banda? 'Well, we were still quite happy here. And I don't think we could have settled into life in England. Anyway, things worked pretty well for a long time. You could get stuff. It was only at the end that it all went wrong. The atmosphere got nasty. But even then, everything was an awful lot better than it is now.'

Friends who visited me sometimes asked if I didn't get depressed by Malaŵi's poverty and refractoriness to development. This would have been a natural reaction, as the country sometimes seemed to become less rather than more functional from one year to the next. The efforts of government and fly-by-night aid agencies made little impact on the prevailing disorder, and faith in progress could be undermined. But although the bigger picture seemed bleak, the example of the Pastimes suggested that, with a different approach, anything might be possible.

I was familiar with the tiny smallholdings of subsistence farmers, their methods changeless since time immemorial. I had also glimpsed monstrous estates dedicated solely to the mass production of cheap tobacco. But the Pastimes supplied a model that was ingenious, small, personal and in harmony with its surroundings. There was of course technical accomplishment, but more important seemed the commitment. They were strangers there and had freely cut their ties with home. It was this that forged their bond with the land and its people, its beauty, hardships and uncertainties.

Only if we learn to dwell can we build; and only if we learn to build can we live with each other, Heidegger observed. I had dabbled in his writings at university, but this observation had little meaning for me until I saw how the Pastimes dwelled on the land alongside their tenants, making the place their home rather than merely living there. It was the proof of T.S. Eliot's claim that 'love of a country begins as attachment to our own field of action'.

When Tom died suddenly, a few years later, Flora drove over to the District Commissioner to report the death.

'I am extremely sorry to hear that, madam. Please accept my condolences.' There was then a pause before he asked: 'Why are you telling me?'

'I thought I was supposed to report it.'

'No, don't worry – you don't have to tell anybody.'

And so Tom was buried in a shallow grave dug by his workers in front of the house, just before the paddock where his favourite horses grazed. I visited a year later to pay my respects.

'You see how the ground's fallen in,' Flora observed matter-of-factly. Indeed, below a small tombstone, an oblong depression in the turf betrayed where the earth had consumed her husband's remains.

I looked all around at the house Tom had built, the woods he had planted, the fields he had sowed, and the lives he had nurtured – and then I tried and failed to recall some lines of Eliot which seemed apt:

> Old stone to new building, old timber to new fires,
> Old fires to ashes, and ashes to the earth
> Which is already flesh, fur and faeces,
> Bone of man and beast, cornstalk and leaf.

One day, perhaps very soon, the Pastimes' efforts would be subsumed. In the broader context of white settlers in Africa, that might be in accordance with historic justice. But it all seemed unimportant at that moment by the grave:

Tom was dwelling forever in the land he loved, equalised, and without incongruity.

XXIX

ON RUINS

In a hidden cleft on a nearby mountain, the Pastimes had once built a cottage, nestled among dusky conifers. It enjoyed a sweeping view over the plain below, with their farm just visible in the far distance. It was small but exquisitely constructed, with a tin roof and timber walls set on a base of hefty stones. All around was a soft dense carpet of pine needles and, behind, a trickling stream was bowered with foliage drooping with berries. An occasional trout lurked beneath banks overhung with wild flowers. The water had been diverted into a narrow channel and thence to a little reservoir behind the building. At night you went to sleep to the sound of its gentle burbling.

The one living area contained bed, easy chairs and dining table, all roughly crafted by hand. At the back was set a stone fireplace, with a tank built into the wall above for hot water. There was no electricity: the kitchen had a paraffin fridge and a cast-iron stove, and the rooms were illumined by candelabra, inventively fashioned from logs that could be lowered from the ceiling by ropes and pulleys. When all were lit, the whole cottage – which was octagonal in shape – glowed like a storm lantern.

I stayed there once – perhaps the most peaceful night I have ever known. I recall the crackling of the fire and the occasional hoot of an owl, the soft glow of embers as I drifted off and the deep orange light of dawn piercing the fir trees to wake me. But when I next visited the Pastimes a few years later, their cottage was gone. They had been struggling to maintain the place, which, with age, they used less and less often. When they did visit, they invariably found the firewood looted. Then the door got smashed in, and panes of glass, utensils and furniture were taken. When the whole tin roof went missing, the interior spoiled with rain. For a time they repaired and replaced everything, even setting watchmen to guard the property, but the battle proved unwinnable.

I went up the mountain to visit the ruin and found the stone base enduring, but everything else lifted or broken, the whole space scattered with shards of broken glass and splintered timber. As I stepped among the debris, I found on the ground the small plaque formerly affixed to the wall beside the front door. Tom had etched on it a haiku by the seventeenth-century Japanese poet Basho:

> Those who see the lightning
> And think nothing:
> How precious they are!

Though I never asked Tom what the words meant to him, they seemed to extol serenity before the forces of destruction.

'There are some good ruins in this country,' I said to Dr Highbrow.

'Yes,' he replied, 'and Malaŵi produces new ones in a very acceptable period of time.'

It was he who first took me to see the ruins of the 'old church' at Mtakataka, built in the 1900s but surrendered to flooding only a decade later. Its missionary architects were not discouraged and simply moved several miles away to Mua – the place where Boucher today presides over his ethnographical museum.

To reach the old church, you have to leave the nearest tarmac road and follow sandy, unpromising-looking tracks, clearly not intended for vehicles, though navigable in the dry season. These lead you through maize fields and scrub to a river, which it is necessary to ford on foot. After this, you trudge for an hour along grassy trails before – suddenly – there flashes above the swaying cornstalks a vision like a celestial city from a mediaeval painting. It is a massive crenellated edifice, complex in style, with Romanesque and pointed arches, hexagonal belfries, Baroque pediment and recesses. But it is very obviously defunct, the interior dense with foliage sprouting from every aperture. Trees have sprung through the roof, and roots creep out of wide gaps in the masonry. At the top of the façade stands a simple wooden cross, but this teeters at a 45-degree angle.

Up close – thanks to a machete to hack through the vegetation – you notice the bricks, which are of rare quality: robust but elaborate, some even shaped in ornamental bevelled moulds, as I have seen nowhere else in Malaŵi. Despite a century of battery by the elements, most are in excellent condition.

By contrast, today's locally fired bricks – the products of smouldering kilns found in every village – are often of woefully poor quality. Whether for want of technique, effort or materials, they lack durability, and dwellings built from them melt away like sand castles after a few rainy seasons. The bricks from the 'old church', though ancient, were therefore highly prized in the vicinity. Gradually they were being hacked from the fabric of the building and recycled into shacks. I visited several times over a period of ten years and, on each occasion, another part of the church had been lost. First the east end disappeared, with its apse and tower. A few years later went the transepts, then the nave. At last, only the façade remained.

In studying Classics, your whole training is a response to ruins. The discipline was first kindled by the excavation of buildings consumed by centuries of dirt, by the discovery of broken statues in fields around the Mediterranean. In Malaŵi, I found myself taking an indecent delight in the opportunity to watch in real time the processes that had reduced the ancient world to rubble. What I observed at Mtakataka had also taken place in Europe in the Dark Ages.

The comparison stirred Dr Highbrow to drive to South Africa for a Classics conference, where he offered a paper on the Roman ruins that endured in Anglo-Saxon England, drawing parallels with ruins in southern Africa. He quoted an anonymous eighth-century poem which, aside from the reference to frost, described well what we saw at Mtakataka:

> Wondrous is this foundation – the fates have broken
> And shattered this city; the work of giants crumbles.
> The roofs are ruined, the towers toppled,
> Frost in the mortar has broken the gate,
> Torn and worn and shorn by the storm,
> Eaten through with age.

The puny huts around Mtakataka made the 'old church' feel like 'giants' work' in just the same way that the Roman ruins had impressed the Anglo-Saxons, who used them as quarries but were unable to produce anything as lasting or substantial. Yet the same response, Dr Highbrow noted, could be found as far back as Ancient Greece, when the citizens of Athens and Alexandria considered older, mightier edifices than their own age knew how to make: the great walls of Mycenae and Tiryns could have been built only by the Cyclopes, they supposed.

Studying the classical world, you are edified by the example of the past, humbled by the inadequacy of the present and dismayed by the reckoning of what has been lost. Simultaneously, there is a great equalising effect: every people has been here before, and even your own forebears once wandered in bafflement among giants' work before emerging from the desolation to create afresh.

But our delight in ruins is complex, ambiguous. Oswald Spengler's unsettling 1918 work, *The Decline of the West*, identified ruins as a peculiarly European obsession, and not necessarily a healthy one. Only Europeans, he observed, insisted on aestheticising what was broken, on preserving objects *in their fallen state*. In the eighteenth and nineteenth centuries, they even went so far as to construct artificial ruins in the form of 'follies' for the adornment of their parks and gardens – an impulse which other cultures would have found perverse. The same feeling could be detected in the preference for patina on antique bronzes. Their original Greek and Roman sculptors would have judged them merely dirty.

Certainly I was aware of some such feeling in myself as I returned again and again to Mtakataka to monitor its disintegration. On my last visit, the teetering wooden cross had fallen, and I found myself lamenting not so much what it stood for but rather the perfect appearance of the ruin as it had been. I would have liked to put the cross back, at a wonky angle, out of a purely aesthetic impulse. Ruins seduce us into idle contemplation, hinting at the sweetness of inaction and the futility of effort.

Yet this predilection seems absurd elsewhere. In Asia I have often been alarmed by the gaudy reconstruction of charming old buildings, the disdain for what is obsolete.

'Eternity should not inhabit the building, but the builder,' observed the sinologist Simon Leys in his essay on the Chinese attitude to the past. Ancient Chinese architecture was perhaps even intended to be impermanent, he suggested: 'the transient nature of the construction is like an offering to the voracity of time; for the price of such sacrifices, the constructors ensure the everlastingness of their spiritual designs'.

Here was a parallel to an abandoned Malaŵian tradition, which decreed the burning of a man's house when he died to mark his transition to 'the village on the other side' – the world of the ancestors. The practice proclaimed an indifference to the merely physical, and a confidence in the durability of the spirit. In all the villages around the old church, children abounded, as they did throughout the country, excitedly greeting the arrival of visitors. Everywhere they pranced numberless and joyful among the puny huts and withering fields, among the feeble brick kilns and the village graveyards. What was important was the connectedness between living, dead and unborn, not a sentimental attachment to the material remains. Unperturbed by the magnificent ruin in their midst, life went on, changeless, fertile and ebullient.

XXX

THE USES OF LITERACY

In the National Museum in Blantyre, I found cleft sticks and calabashes, cowrie currency and bark cloth suits, ivory nose plugs, fanciful percussion instruments, brass coils for the adornment of limbs – a fine collection, with everything ordered, labelled, sensibly displayed. But the life was gone from it all, and, when I visited, I was the sole person there. Only a collection of witches' charms, fashioned from beads, pods and pieces of string, still suggested a certain maleficent potential. Everything else was defunct and shrouded in dust. Some Nyau masks nestled in a corner, looking particularly forlorn, their fabric crumpled and rotting, the elaborate manes of feather and sisal limp and desiccated. You might have mistaken one for a small dead animal beginning to decompose.

The more sensitive Westerners in Malaŵi were aware that their modernity could soon corrode the local culture, which many worked hard to conserve in museums such as this one. But attempts to curate can themselves be deadening; indeed, the interest of the ethnographer is almost pathognomonic of a culture in peril.

An earlier Nyau tradition insisted that the masks be burnt after each performance and constructed anew for the next, just like the houses of the deceased. It was the very opposite of curation, suggesting supreme confidence in the creative power of the mask-maker, in the vitality of his culture, and in the primacy of the message over the artefact.

I don't believe Sangala burnt his masks, though the dancing at his village had nevertheless been fulsome, even ugly, and very much alive. I was lucky to live in one of the districts of Malaŵi in which the tradition still flourished; elsewhere, it was fading from existence. Occasionally *gule* was filmed and broadcast on Malaŵian television, which seemed almost to confirm the decay of the art form. The assurance of digital eternity provided a licence to ignore it – just as it does when gallery visitors in Europe wander among Titians and Rembrandts and pause only to snap them with their cameras.

Conservation falters when it focuses on the material remains while neglecting their animating spirit. That spirit is of course elusive and intangible, but Thomas Cullen Young, a missionary-ethnographer from Scotland, saw literacy – and then literature – as the means to capture, communicate and renew it in Malaŵi. In this vision, he had a profound influence on Kamuzu Banda.

Literacy was still an innovation in the country when Cullen Young arrived in 1904. Local peoples had until recently been almost entirely letterless and, even among Muslim tribes, what was known of the Koran was preserved mainly through memory and recitation. Malaŵi is home to various rock-art sites, which testify, as elsewhere, to man's deep-seated need to record his experiences for posterity. Some are surprisingly new, with cave paintings even of cars and helicopters, but most are older and depict hunting scenes, tribal ritual, *gule wamkulu*. But any deeper meaning is inscrutable, and the images are eloquent mainly of the limits of communication without the written word.

The teaching of literacy became central to missionary

endeavour, and Cullen Young in particular was passionate about this task. It was in his classroom that he first encountered Banda – though the significance of that meeting was not immediately apparent.

It is a remarkable story: in 1940, having retired back to Scotland, Cullen Young noticed an African passer-by in the street near a university building in Edinburgh. The two made eye contact and began a conversation in which each was surprised to discover in the other an intimate knowledge of Kasungu District, Malaŵi. Here was Banda, who had just moved over from America.

Cullen Young did not recognise him, but Banda most certainly remembered Cullen Young, though he did not say so. Only later, when their friendship was firmly established, would he choose to stir the older man's memories of the mission school where he had taught thirty years before, and of a pupil there who jostled and defied the teacher's instructions to remain seated – though this, Banda explained, was only because he had been too short to read the blackboard from the back of the class. Cullen Young had become exasperated and expelled the boy, who then set off on a long journey on foot to find education elsewhere. Banda bore no grudge, and now, decades on, their friendship blossomed as they collaborated on linguistic, literary and anthropological projects.

From different perspectives, they shared a concern for the upheaval of African culture by modernity. They lamented how ancient ways were increasingly discredited by Western know-how. Old hierarchies were being displaced by new ones, and commerce and development lured people from their homes and each other. The purpose of education in Africa, Cullen Young insisted, must be to redress this loss, 'to fulfil, not destroy' the indigenous culture.

Central to village life was the 'talking-place' – the

mphara – where young and old traditionally convened, in the presence of the ancestors, to discuss the issues facing the community. It was a vital institution, Cullen Young noted, the analogue of forum and agora, parliament and senate. But it had begun to vanish from the societies he observed, so he founded a local-language newspaper with the explicit object of creating a new forum for discussion, adapted to the times. By 'throwing its columns open to the African contributor', the newspaper would become the 'equal property of all concerned'.

Cullen Young also supported literary competitions, and encouraged and compiled the work of upcoming Malaŵian writers. Perhaps the most moving project was a collaboration with Banda to sponsor and edit an anthology of the country's heritage. *Our African Way of Life* is an attempt to preserve the memories of 'the last [Malaŵians] to have personal touch with the past; the last for whom the word "grandmother" will mean some actually remembered person who could speak of a time when the land of the Lake knew no white man'. As Cullen Young and Banda explained, the writers were all motivated by 'a simple love and pride for their African ways of thought and their people's mode of life': 'Conscious of the impact of a civilisation which considers itself superior [. . .] they are none of them prepared at all points to admit that superiority [. . .] They try – while yet there is time: while still the old they value is in being – to get through to the European mind some inkling of their African truth, their African scale of values, their African social ethic.'

The first author they championed, John Kambalame, was a soldier in the British army, who had written his essay in 1942, while fighting the Japanese in the Far East. He had a sustaining vision of home and wanted urgently to communicate it. He wrote about the making of a good household, the raising of children, participation in the life of the village, rites of passage. Kambalame feared his people were discarding their culture because of the allure of another, and so wanted to impress upon the young 'what [was] good among our ancient ways': 'those things which were understood long ago and belong to [our] own people. Thereafter they will combine them with the things they are being taught today. Having done that, they will receive the thanks of both parties [. . .] because of their rightly using both old and new together.'

In this shared project, Kambalame, Cullen Young and Banda hoped that literature might revitalise the culture fading around them. In this, there is a parallel with the work of another, more famous, writer from the other side of the continent: Chinua Achebe. With his great trilogy, the Nigerian novelist would recount the disintegration of a tribal society over successive generations. In the first novel, *Things Fall Apart*, a contented and self-sufficient Igbo community, bound tight by ancient lore, is destroyed by the arrival of the British, who, the narrator tells, 'put a knife to the things that held us together, and now we have fallen apart'. The following novels are a painful study in the disjunction of Western and African cultures.

Achebe wrote in a high and sensitive style, with constant reference to European literature. His title comes of course from *The Second Coming*, Yeats's premonitory vision of the end of civilisation, but the novel also alludes to T.S. Eliot, A.E. Housman and the King James version. His references to the Western canon are variously playful, affectionate and critical, but when you are so intertwined with a tradition, you become a part of it.

'The stranglehold of English Lit,' wrote Malawian poet Felix Mnthali, was 'the heart of alien conquest'. It was once a fashionable view: that literature was an insidious weapon in the arsenal of cultural imperialism. But Achebe's trilogy suggests a more astute response. As cultural commingling and cultural decline are inevitable, there can be 'no going back'; yet writing may supply a way forward. Literature becomes a tool for salvaging something of Achebe's own threatened heritage. In adapting the Western novel to tell an African story, two clashing traditions may thus renew one another.

Achebe was strict about his method: 'Those who do the work of extending the frontiers of English so as to accommodate African thought-patterns must do it through their mastery of English and not out of innocence.' It is a sentiment I can imagine being heartily endorsed by Banda. First things first. To write about Africa, you must study English. To study English, you need Latin. For Latin, Greek – and so on. 'An education without Classics is a house built on sand!' Before Classics – 'learn your own ways first!' Grammar and correct usage. History and culture, African and European. Julius Caesar and tribal lore. It feels like a *reductio ad absurdum* of Achebe's position – but the same sincere impulse is at work.

Banda's obsession with ancient languages, and the extravagance of Kamuzu Academy – that 'Eton of Africa' – can appear perverse from a European perspective but must also be understood as expressions of pride and excitement in the spread of the written word. The supreme symbol of this was the University of Malaŵi and, especially, Chancellor College, which opened as a centre for the humanities in 1973. It was the fulfilment of perhaps Banda's most youthful dream: that the highest education, even in the arts, might be made available to his own people, within their own country. It was at this university that his wilder ambition – of a Malaŵian literary tradition – would also be realised. But literature is unpredictable and politically intractable. When it blossomed in Malaŵi, it was not what Banda had in mind.

Chancellor's is a magnificent building from that odd phase of mid twentieth-century architecture which managed to make so much more of African settings than of European ones. Exposed cement and steel are discordant but still somehow beautiful against the woods and foothills of Zomba. The severe lines of Brutalist cloisters are softened by foliage, and the grey walls offset by the abundant red and purple of flame trees and jacarandas. The auditorium, an imposing, jagged, hexagonal structure, tapers outwards like the conning tower of an aircraft carrier.

Nearby, Kamuzu Banda's opening of the university is commemorated on a massive bronze plaque in a clear bold script. Only if you stand very close can you read four other words, carved in minute, lowercase lettering, at the bottom edge: *'exegi monumentum aere perennius'*.

It is the most famous line of the Roman poet Horace, who wrote in the first century BC: 'I have left a monument more lasting than bronze.' The claim is meant to apply to his poetry, to the immortality of literature; however, the line has been misappropriated by megalomaniacs down the ages to assert their glory. It would be easy to imagine a dictator such as Banda using the quotation in just this way – except, why was the lettering so tiny? A friend who taught at the university noted that not one of his students realised the words were there until he pointed them out. It is hard to see bombast in such unobtrusive, almost secretive, use of the quotation.

To my mind, this small detail reveals that Banda was alive to the frailty of his monument and the words' real meaning. The grandiosity of Horace's claim no doubt had its appeal for him as well, but at base he knew the poet was right: that writing alone assured continuity, that the physical traces must vanish. It was an invitation, maybe a challenge to the members of his university to create something that would outlast the buildings.

Indeed, from the late 1960s onwards, Malaŵians discovered an enthusiasm for high literature that would have astonished Cullen Young and the authors of the anthology on which he and Banda had collaborated. Novelists, playwrights, essayists and, especially, poets began to proliferate around a core based at the university. Frank Chipasula was the first to be published, and Jack Mapanje perhaps the best known, but there were many others. They called themselves the Malaŵi Writers Group, and their first anthology, *Mau*, extolling the beauty of their country, its people and its myths, was published in 1971. Educated Malaŵians began to adopt *belles lettres* as something of a national pastime. Another poet, Steve Chimombo, more recently produced a directory of the country's writers, and its catalogue of published poets runs to twenty-nine pages. Has anywhere else in Africa produced such a flowering from so small a population?

In the 1970s, as Banda became more authoritarian, the poets became more political, more dissident. Whether intentionally or not, they developed into a nucleus of resistance to the regime, and their confidence and numbers grew almost in proportion to government efforts to suppress them. The criticism was at first cautious, encrypted in an elaborate system of literary code, as when Mapanje used classical allusion to suggest that Malaŵi was like Thebes under Creon, the tyrant from Sophocles' *Antigone*. But the hostility was soon detected, with persecution following swiftly and mercilessly. Chipasula was driven into exile, along with David Rubadiri, Lupenga Mphande and Paul Zeleza. Countless others suffered bullying, intimidation and censorship. Felix Mnthali and Jack Mapanje – who were both professors at the university – were imprisoned without charge and held in barbarous conditions.

They responded with poetry that was visceral and acerbic but deeply sensitive, rich in literary reference and powerfully uplifting, as when Mnthali, in his poem 'December Seventh, 'Seventy-six', described his own incarceration but also the possibility of consolation in even such harrowing circumstances:

> PERCHED on a bucket of faeces
> Freshly cleansed of its night-soil
> I brood on the simplicity of man
> While all around me stand
> Throngs of faces
> Faces in knots of ten or more
> Glued to the vibrations of other faces
> > Wrinkled
> > Wizened
> > Pained
> Beyond their years and hanging on bodies
> That once looked human
> Clutching with iron hands
> Filthy plates of lukewarm porridge
> Without sugar and without salt
> AND HOLDING FORTH
> On history
> On politics
> On Shakespeare
> On tea-growing
> On engineering
> On metaphysics
> On pragmatism
> On existentialism . . .

> On witches' brews and
> Miraculous escapes from prison [. . .]
> On anecdotes of conquest and
> Feats of seduction
> For discussion kept us warm
> > In these dead surroundings

Mnthali was released after four months, but Mapanje was in prison for almost four years. He requested a skipping rope for exercise, but was refused, and this came to symbolise all the many other deprivations he suffered – including that of pen and paper. Yet his guards could not stop him composing poetry in his head, committing it to memory. And so 'Skipping Without Rope' became a metaphor for his spirit rising above repression.

> I do, you don't, I can, you can't,
>
> I will, you won't, I see, you don't, I
> Sweat, you don't, I will, will wipe my
> Gluey brow then wipe you at a stroke
> I will, will wipe your horrid, stinking,
>
> Vulgar prison rules, will wipe you all
> Then hop about, hop about my cell, my
> Home, the mountains, my globe as your
> Sparrow hops about your prison yard
>
> Without your hope, without your rope,
> I swear, I will skip without your rope

Mapanje became one of Malaŵi's most famous 'prisoners of conscience', a beacon of resistance to dictatorship in Africa. A long campaign for his release was fought by

Amnesty and PEN International, supported by writers and activists from Wole Soyinka to Diane Abbott. Harold Pinter read Mapanje's poems at a protest outside the Malaŵi High Commission in London. When staff at the University of Edinburgh wrote directly to Banda, he was stirred to answer his alma mater, but remained unmoved: Mapanje was 'subversive' so he had to be 'picked out and detained [. . .] This is Malaŵi in Africa and not another country. Things have to be done according to the conditions and circumstances in Malaŵi, Africa', the letter concluded stiffly. But mightier political forces were gathering: the Cold War had ended, Mandela had just been released, and Western governments suddenly became less tolerant of allies whose regimes now tarnished the victory of democracy. Mapanje was set free in 1991.

The ironies are bittersweet. Banda had once sought to foster a literary tradition in Malaŵi; he even sowed the seeds. But when one sprang up before him, he was like Caliban enraged at the mirror and could think only of how to destroy it. Yet he failed: Malaŵi's poets were 'well-equipped', wrote Frank Chipasula. They possessed 'the Word: the vocabulary necessary to name the wrong'. Against this, Banda's brutality proved powerless and in fact stimulated greater eloquence and vitality, which, when he was younger, might have drawn his admiration.

Would Malaŵian literature exist without him? His contribution, as with so much else, seems ambiguous, inadvertent, but also indispensable. He got his monument more lasting than bronze. He could not see it; it defied and indicted him; but it also proved – triumphantly – the power of the written word to surprise and endure.

PART FOUR

THE NEED FOR ROOTS

XXXI

MODERN TIMES

Banda's new capital city Lilongwe was founded in 1971, with impressive showpiece structures constructed in the same ultra-modern style as the university: the Reserve Bank is spaceship-like, an inverted pyramid with a tessellated surface of tiles, recesses and slit windows. State House, like a bold abstract painting, is a grid of unadorned columns and flagpoles intersecting with blank concrete oblongs suspended weightlessly above airy courtyards. The modernity strikes a defiant, optimistic note as it confronts the dusty wilderness all around.

Unfortunately only a core of administrative buildings and main roads resulted from the original masterplan; the rest of the city was just left to happen. As its population snowballed, Lilongwe became an immense sprawl of flimsy clutter, with only islands of solidity and order to remind you of Banda's grand design.

Much of the population lives in cramped suburban slums, densely packed with structures of mud brick and salvaged plywood, rusted tin sheets and dirty tarpaulin. I passed through these periodically on my way in and out of the city, but sometimes had to pause longer, as when searching for used auto-parts. My mechanic Mussa led me on a number of frenetic quests to find items out of stock in the city's main suppliers. Such missions could extend over several days, as we visited a succession of vendors and sifted through their wares, which were usually jumbled up in torn and grease-smeared plastic bags. The grimy valves and gaskets, bolts and bushes would be tipped onto the dirt floor, and I would defer to Mussa to pick through these with his fingers, in the hope of chancing upon what was needed.

Waiting in the car, I surveyed the cruel scene around me. The air was hazy and stank of refuse, diesel fumes, wood-smoke and burning plastic from the firepits where children played and scavenged. Everything was painfully compressed, homes cheek-by-jowl with workshops and rubbish heaps. Childcare and light industry were conducted side by side: a young mother was breastfeeding in the welder's yard; a girl carried her baby sister on her back as she went about the work of touting plastic bags. Another minded her family's potato-chip stall, snarling at the young men who teetered from the boozing parlour to harass her.

Children everywhere were absorbed in work, however demeaning. They begged for near worthless coins and empty bottles, or sat beside the mechanic's shop, picking apart ruined tyres into threads of rubber that could be sold as twine. A few young girls loitered at the roadside, their clothes scanty, their eyes without innocence, assessed coldly by a trio of haulage drivers who stood by their lorries sharing a cigarette. On a patch of dusty wasteland, an emaciated cowherd was driving three emaciated cows among strands of parched grass sprouting between tangles of charred wire and discarded scrap metal. One recalcitrant animal ignored the boy's stick and continued to graze behind the rest. I watched as he clumped wearily over to pick up a rock, which he then flung at the animal's flank. It bounced off, the cow did not even flinch, and the boy resumed his futile thrashing.

My attention was drawn to a breeze-block shell patched with uneven timbers and plastic sheeting. It seemed the focus of considerable interest, so I sauntered over. The deafening thud of amplifiers came from within, loud enough to be heard above the clamour of motor horns and car breakers. It was a cinema, guarded by intimidating bouncers at the entrance. I peered inside, where men were packed as into a crowded prison cell. The room had a rancid odour, but the occupants seemed accepting of this as they stared intently at the screen, which showed a dismemberment scene from a grotesque American gangster film.

'Thousand kwachas, big man,' one of the bouncers offered. I declined, so he turned his attention to the children who had clambered up the sides to peep through gaps beneath the tarpaulin roof. One by one they were plucked from their vantage positions and tossed roughly to the floor.

I returned to my car to wait for Mussa and remembered a comment from the book in Banda's library about colonial administration from the 1930s. The author recounted how he was sometimes asked to explain why Africans degenerated when they lived in cities. The question was fallacious, he retorted. In his view, *all* people degenerated when they lived in cities, black and white. Europeans were just heedless of the effect on themselves.

In Lilongwe, everywhere teemed with people so that you could imagine no neighbourhood existing there, only more or less unfamiliar faces in the immense throng of passing strangers. Against the happy communality I knew from almost everywhere else in Malaŵi, this was a perversion of the village ideal.

At length and to my relief, Mussa emerged, glowing with triumph and holding high a worn and insignificant-looking piece of metal. We had then to settle a price with its vendor, who was already drunk at eleven in the morning.

It was an interesting negotiation, in which both sides had to acknowledge that this item of refuse was of inestimable value to me, but at the same time almost worthless to anyone else. Mussa and he shook hands on a price of about ten pounds, and the vendor thanked him profusely.

'*Zikomo*, big man!'

'Big man' is a common honorific in Malaŵi, and in the slums it seemed to be conferred on anyone who did not have the misfortune to live there. In less wretched circles, however, it denoted a particular class: Big Men are the few who have made it, whose wealth is of a different order of magnitude to any that could be dreamt of by the majority of the population.

Big Men live in mansions and ride in limousines. They consort in hotel lobbies and can afford foreign travel. They may have assets abroad and the security that confers. They need never go hungry. Indeed 'Big Man' can be understood quite literally: the inequality in wealth is so vast that it results in inequality even in physical size between the elite and the poor. Between them, the gulf lies all but empty: Malaŵi's middle class is conspicuously small and seems to a great extent the confection of foreign aid agencies who employ local staff. The economy is tiny, with few resources and little commerce. The great source of wealth is foreign aid, almost a third of the country's GDP when I lived there. Opportunity to tap into this was a major determinant of personal prosperity.

As I drove out of the slum, the dirt track turned to tarmac, lined for a stretch by a series of enormous frames for billboard advertisements, all empty. The scaffolds loomed like skeletons until we passed a single hoarding with a vast image of President Bingu wa Mutharika in a turquoise jump suit and cowboy hat. He was laying bricks, and the slogan read: 'Let the work of my hands speak for itself!'

Bingu was Malaŵi's third president, elected in 2004. He had succeeded Bakili Muluzi, a wheeler-dealer with a conviction for theft and a reputation for black-marketeering who had risen to the cabinet under Banda before setting up his own party. Muluzi was the champion of the 'multi-party democracy' that saw the end of Banda's regime, and he promised a new era of liberalism and affluence.

The country breathed a sigh of relief, as a myriad of petty constraints were lifted. Banda's 'Four Pillars' of society – Loyalty, Obedience, Unity, Discipline – were mocked and discarded. The obsession with modesty in dress and behaviour seemed stuffy and irrelevant. Ancient village hierarchies, once championed by Banda, began to lose their prestige. Television was introduced in 1996.

There was something of an 'I'm alright, Jack' atmosphere to this period. Muluzi's administration quickly became notorious for corruption. As the government's coffers emptied, the Big Men got richer, economic decline gathered pace, the dysfunctionality spread. I was astonished to uncover evidence of the infrastructure which once existed in Malaŵi: railways, lake vessels, a national airline, manufacturing and retail, investment by multi-national corporations. When I lived in the country, I could never have imagined these once existed, although I do recall a disused railway line with a mature baobab thrusting up between the tracks. The decay started in the last decade of Banda's rule, but real disintegration came in the years that followed.

In 1998, Muluzi sold the entire national grain reserve a year before the worst famine in recent history. The money from the sale was never fully accounted for, and the people starved to death in their thousands. In the ensuing outrage,

Muluzi was succeeded by Bingu, who was president when I arrived in 2009.

For a while, things seemed to go better under his administration, which was certainly slicker. If there was embezzlement, it was not so flagrant as to endanger the supply of foreign aid. Yet there was a hollowness to politics after Banda. All the parties claimed to stand for democracy, but there seemed little to choose from between the Democratic Progressive Party, the United Democratic Front, the Alliance for Democracy, the People's Party . . . They were all just congregations gathering behind rival Big Men in hope of patronage if their chief attained office. It was a new tribalism. There were no differing political principles, neither left nor right, socialist, liberal or conservative. The Big Men just had their regional power bases and blocs of supporters, united in expectation of largesse following victory. Political campaigning might even take the form of Big Men riding in motorcades through villages, tossing handfuls of low denomination currency at the wretched – an image evocative of the late Roman Republic at its nadir.

Once office was attained, the most important task was to encourage the flow of aid money into the country, and Bingu was initially adroit at this. Indeed, he did so while also maintaining a posture of independence and self-respect. He made much of his vision for a river port in the south intended to connect Malaŵi to the Indian Ocean. Vast sums were put up for this, but it was not even half-finished before the whole project was left to ruin. Nevertheless, the money showed no sign of drying up: in fact, Bingu was by now being courted by the People's Republic of China which, in 2010, paid for an ugly new parliament building and an immense hotel and conference centre, named in his honour. He was about to take his turn as chairman of the Organisation of African Unity, and the centre was designed to anticipate the exalted diplomacy that would ensue. One of his acolytes commented that only Bingu had the far-sightedness to invest in important infrastructure such as this.

When I arrived in the country, Bingu was ascendant, and there had been no egregious misrule. To use Dr Highbrow's phrase, I was adjusting well to 'what passes for normality in Malaŵi'. That was all about to change.

XXXII

SPEECH DAYS

The psychedelic quality of life at Kamuzu Academy was most powerful on Founder's Day. Various Big Men from parliament, the judiciary and the diplomatic corps would attend to make speeches and give prizes. The higher the status of the guest of honour, the greater the spectacle. There might be a welcoming party comprised of uniformed police and soldiery; regiments of women, swaying and chanting; corpulent dark-suited ministers; Lords Spiritual, cassocked, surpliced and tippeted in crimson and mauve; Paramount Chiefs in gay apparel; 'Traditional Authorities', District Commissioners, Chief Justices, Right Honourables and Excellencies.

Children and staff had already assembled on a wide expanse of lawn in all their splendour. At the vanguard, head boy and head girl held aloft the school's and the nation's standards while, behind them, straw boaters and brass buttons shimmered on a dense regiment of pupils. Among the masters, the colourful hoods and gowns, caps and tassels of diverse African universities eclipsed the sub fusc of British degree holders, at least until the appearance of Dr Highbrow, his purple and scarlet DPhil robes unfurled. This procession then marched slowly through the grounds towards the clock-tower, to the cheers and wonderment of a vast crowd of onlookers. But formation was broken as the column reached the bottleneck into the Great Hall, so that pupils and masters, bishops and dancing girls, sergeants and servants of state and doctors of philosophy were jumbled pell-mell as the cavalcade of black Mercedes rolled up at the porte-cochère to deliver the Big Man.

Waiting is an important part of the occasion and, for the most important guests, you wait very long indeed. We in fact waited all morning on the day the academy was visited by President Bingu himself. His approach was advertised by the wail and screech of police cars and fire trucks, followed by the growing thud of rotors: the president arrived in not one but two helicopters. What great favour the school had been shown, the chaplain was heard to remark, by such obvious extravagance. Lesser Big Men fussed and fretted around Bingu as he moved ponderously from his aircraft to the auditorium. As he took his place on the dais, there came a deafening crash of amplified percussion as Mr Chisomo, the director of music, clad in a gold suit, opened the proceedings with his own arrangement of the 'Hallelujah Chorus'. Bingu had just been re-elected, and he signalled his approval of this welcome by demanding an encore.

There followed a long presidential address on 'bright futures' and the price of cement, fertiliser subsidies and the importance of 'dreaming in colour'. 'The proof of the pudding is in the eating,' Bingu pronounced on the sagacity of his economic policies. 'And now – we are eating the pudding!' Rapturous applause. 'And it tastes good!' The audience rose to its feet, and 'Oi-eiii Bingu! Bingu oi-eiii!' thundered antiphonically round the hall.

Afterwards, Bingu took a tour of inspection and was invited to observe a model lesson, given by Dr Highbrow on the historian Thucydides. The dignitaries assembled at the front of the classroom to hear him speak in words somewhat like these: 'The Athenians are at war with Sparta.

Their first casualties are given a public funeral. Pericles delivers the oration, but uses it to celebrate the ideals of the city: "First honour your ancestors – they are the source of your wealth and freedom. But you should not hanker for the past. Athenians are innovators. Pioneers of democracy and justice. The envy of the world in all the arts of war and peace."

'At that moment, victory felt assured. But like a tragedian, Thucydides sets this speech on the eve of catastrophe. Athens is at the tense moment of apogee.' Dr Highbrow chalked a parabola on the blackboard. The real lesson of Thucydides is –'

Bingu had waited patiently on Dr Highbrow's grandiloquence, but now he rose to interrupt its flow. There were smiles of thanks, low murmurs of approval, handshakes and expansive gestures. He made for his helicopter, the heavy entourage following him out.

The Chinese ambassador attended the following year. Relations between the two countries were being consummated after Bingu had ended diplomatic recognition of Taiwan six months before. The ambassador cut a handsome figure in smart grey pinstripe, with an improbable spray of violets in his buttonhole. He spoke softly and slowly, so at first I thought the pupils would grow restless. But his delivery was deliberate, charismatic, even portentous, and the audience were soon captured: 'China is both big and small. She is young and she is old. Modern and ancient. She is rich and she is poor. China . . .'

After half an hour he lavishly rewarded their attention. At his signal, the doors at the far end were flung open, and a train of bearers staggered the length of the hall with crates of laptops and stereos, racquets and trainers, keyboards and plastic recorders, illustrated histories and Chinese textbooks. The whoops and cheers grew deafening as, crate by crate, the treasure was unloaded at the ambassador's feet. With some difficulty, he prevailed for a moment's silence to announce his final offering: a pair of Mandarin teachers and an annual university scholarship to the People's Republic. The audience erupted into frenzy.

How different was the visit of Britain's High Commissioner a year later. An unprepossessing figure in a crumpled suit, he arrived – it was well noted – not with a string of limousines but in a solitary Japanese pick-up. He delivered a rambling homily on the various development projects Her Majesty's Government was involved with. He spoke of 'commitments . . . obligations . . . responsibilities . . . the wrongs of the past', but managed to make it all sound like a painful, thankless duty. He even solemnly disclaimed the legacy of colonialism, but his audience had already lost interest and began muttering impatiently.

'Above all define standards, prescribe values', wrote Felix Mnthali sarcastically in 'Neocolonialism', a poem addressed to those who vie for power in Africa:

> And even if you have no satellites in space
> And no weapons of any value
> You will rule the world . . .
> Whatever tune you sing
> They will dance [. . .]
> And you may well pick
> And choose
> Their rare minerals
> And their rich forests
> Prescribe values
> And define standards
> And then sit back
> To allow the third world
> To fall into your lap

Published in 1982, it was an incisive observation at a time when Africa's former masters mysteriously preserved their influence on the continent, despite losing the clout to back it up. But after those two speech days, I found Mnthali's voice anachronistic, even quaint, suggesting a subtler era when moral authority alone could be imagined to hold sway in the world. 'Defining standards, prescribing values' is notoriously what the Chinese have disavowed in their approach to Africa, but their agenda advances no less efficiently for that.

The British, by contrast, seemed somehow undecided about their purpose in the country. Where China freely indulged, Britain hesitantly censured, torn between meddling and stepping back, as if struggling to kick old parental habits. Bingu had recently bought himself a private jet, so to punish this act of naughtiness, the British cut the aid budget – though only by a fraction of the actual cost of the plane. Relations were therefore already strained when a real scandal broke. Just after the High Commissioner's visit to the academy, an internal memo was leaked from his office, describing the president as 'increasingly autocratic and intolerant of criticism'. Bingu was outraged, and there followed a belligerent exchange which culminated in the High Commissioner's expulsion from the country. Bingu addressed himself to the BBC: far from being 'intolerant', he was 'the most tolerant person you have ever met'. A few weeks later, Britain suspended all aid to Malaŵi, and other Western donors followed suit.

XXXIII

THINGS FALL APART

I spent July and August – winter in Malaŵi – on an extended trip around the south of the country, living mostly out of the back of a Land Rover. The weather was cool, dry and bright, with crisp seasonal winds stirring up a haze from the dusty landscape.

I set off just as international aid had been severed, and there were already forex shortages, the first manifestation of impending catastrophe. The kwacha is a non-convertible currency so cannot be exchanged outside Malaŵi. A friend had spent two days in the capital trying banks and *bureaux de change* for cash to travel abroad. He returned with the princely sum of nine US dollars, his bank advising him they could order no more. Like anyone who could, I stockpiled fuel. A couple of other colleagues began converting their savings into cement and fertiliser.

Meanwhile, Bingu was rolling out a new national flag. In 1964, Banda had chosen a rising sun on a tricolour of red, green and black. Bingu felt this did not adequately represent the current epoch of triumph and prosperity, and had the image redesigned to show the sun fully risen. This necessitated changes to uniforms, passports, vehicle number plates and driving licences, all of which needed incorporation of the new design. The government was much exercised with this costly logistical challenge as the country drifted towards disaster.

As a foreigner, I could observe these developments with detachment, and set off blithely into the wilderness with a few friends. We ascended Mount Mulanje, a gigantic plateau in the south and the country's highest peak. We reached the summit on Bastille Day, marking the occasion with wine and good cheer around a fire in a mountain hut. It was bitterly cold, but we stepped out into the night and, from our elevated position, found that fog had settled in a dense layer over the rest of the plateau below us. Various peaks broke through its flatness to resemble islands in a calm white lake, glowing in the moonlight.

We descended a few days later to discover that pressure on the government had intensified. Friends warned us that fuel and imported goods were becoming scarce. The kwacha was devalued by ten per cent, without effect, and then by a further thirty per cent. It made no difference: the currency was in free fall. A politician had died in circumstances widely regarded as suspicious. Several ministers had been dismissed, accused of treachery. Bingu, whose allies were deserting him, publicly likened their crimes to Lucifer's betrayal of God. He spoke on the radio of 'smoking out' his enemies, and called upon his supporters to enforce discipline 'by whatever means'.

Perhaps unwisely, we proceeded to a wildlife reserve and spent several days without phone signal, feeling more at ease for our distance from the mounting chaos outside. We would rise early and slink about the park in the half-light, hoping to catch sight of game. Many of the animals favoured that hour to visit the river for their morning ablutions, and so, parked amid the undergrowth, we would watch from my car as elephant, antelope and buffalo emerged from the forest to drink and bathe. It felt intensely primordial, with traces of mist rising from the surface of the water in the emergent sunlight. Steam escaped from the nostrils of hippos otherwise submerged, just as it did from our lips as we warmed our hands with our breath. Then, as the sun climbed higher, the animals returned to their hides and we to our camp, there to huddle around wood-fired braziers laden with cauldrons of tea and porridge.

We still had a few jerry-cans of diesel in the back of the car, but not quite enough to get home. When we emerged from the park and stopped at a rural filling station, we found the tanks were empty. The lone attendant told us of disorder in nearby Blantyre, where motorists had been queuing for fuel for days, sleeping overnight in lines of cars that stretched miles down otherwise empty streets. When a single consignment of fuel did arrive, it was depleted almost immediately, despite increasingly strict rationing. It was the same story elsewhere, and rumours hurtled round the country whenever fuel trucks were spotted on the road network. Intense speculation would follow as to which depots they might be headed for. A little fuel was available on the black market, but it was commanding prices of ten dollars a litre or more, and was often diluted. Commerce had come to a standstill, and now severe drug shortages were being reported. Frustration grew and then erupted in violence. The day before, angry mobs had formed and begun rioting and looting in Malaŵi's three biggest cities. We were advised to give them a wide berth, though I was able to drop my companions on the outskirts of Blantyre, where they had decided to stay with friends.

The phone network was still just about working, and I made contact with some South Africans smuggling fuel from Mozambique via back roads in another national park. Now travelling alone, my journey there was eerie: I drove for hours along ordinarily busy roads, passing only half a dozen other vehicles before I reached their camp, which lay at the fringes of an immense forest stretching across the border. Tents raised high on stilts kept you out of the way of elephants and hyenas prowling beneath at night. From these you could glimpse stirrings in the surrounding bush and crocodiles sunning themselves on the banks of the nearby stream.

I had arrived late in the afternoon, and the South Africans were gathered with beers around the campfire, gossiping about the crisis. The violence was escalating; eighteen people had been killed by government forces, who were confronting rioters in Lilongwe and Blantyre with live ammunition. A town in the north had been surrendered to the mob, who then set it on fire. That evening another visitor arrived, having been forced to change direction on his way home from work. He had got as far as the nearest town but had then had to turn back when his car was pelted with stones at a barricade. We traded Cassandra prophecies late into the night, drinking dry the supply of box wine, South African brandy and nauseating Amarula cream liquor.

I felt queasy the next morning and was grateful when one of the camp staff gallantly sucked diesel down a hosepipe to create a siphon, filling my car from one of the gigantic fuel drums smuggled across the border. I was about to begin the long journey home when I heard from another friend who had got stuck visiting the capital. He was an Australian volunteer worker who lived near the academy and had travelled to Lilongwe by bus a week before only to find there was now no transport of any description entering or leaving the city. Impelled by curiosity and recklessness, I decided to pick him up on my way home.

The roads were now even more desolate. I was soon on the M1, the country's main north–south thoroughfare, but even so I passed no other traffic besides an occasional police or army vehicle, and a single black government limousine scuttling in the opposite direction. I began to grow nervous and stopped at a large police training college in case I could glean some information. I had been there once before and found it heaving with staff. That day it was like a ghost-town, with only a couple of cooks and cleaners loitering about. Eventually I found the single officer on duty. She told me that everybody else had been deployed elsewhere. She didn't know if I could even get into the city as many of the roads were barricaded. She tried to ring a colleague, but the mobile network was now down. It was up to me, she said. But if I wanted to try, I would have to hurry as a curfew would be enforced at sundown.

I felt the same giddy rush of foolhardiness and set off again. I was about fifty miles from the capital when something strange happened. The road briefly took me above a village and, looking down on it, I watched as it was swept through by a small tornado – the only one I ever saw in Malaŵi. A market was being held when the dirty grey vortex whirled through, upsetting the stands and sucking the produce up into the air. The distressed villagers flapped helplessly as their goods were scattered far and wide by this bizarre visitor. I drove on, unsettled by the omen.

A few miles outside the city, I was halted at a police barricade. Razor wire had been laid between oil drums weighted down with rocks, and there were armed police and soldiers gathered in throngs. Parked beside the road was an armoured car and, behind it, a pickup truck full of young men armed with assault rifles. They were all wearing blue T-shirts with the insignia of Bingu's Democratic Popular Party. A lad in sunglasses was sharpening panga knives on the tarmac. Two policemen questioned me and inspected my papers. They seemed unsure about letting me pass, but then the armoured car and pickup began to pull off in the direction of town. I was hurriedly beckoned to follow them.

I cleaved tightly to those vehicles as they made their way through the city, empty and wrecked. We passed another police convoy, but saw no one else. The streets were littered with burnt-out cars, a few turned upside down. Shopfronts were smashed in, buildings gutted by fire. There was debris everywhere, and the tarmac here and there had scorch marks where flaming barricades had burnt themselves out. Some heaps of old tyres were still smouldering acridly in the middle of the road.

We reached the crossroads where I had to turn left for the lodge where my friend was sheltering. My escort carried straight on, and I gestured broadly to them to indicate I was parting company. They waved cheerily back at me, and I thankfully completed the last mile or two of my journey without incident.

My friend had passed a fretful day listening to sporadic bursts of automatic gunfire. He was staying in a backpacker lodge in a gated compound, and at one point a mob had fled past the perimeter fence, pursued by paramilitaries into a township further down the road. Word had it the insurrection was quelled. There was still an occasional rattle of firearms during the night, but it was mostly peaceful. The next day it was announced that order had been restored. Bingu was clinging on, though apparently only by a thread. He had appealed widely for support but with minimal success, his friend Robert Mugabe obliging with a few consignments of fuel that did little to ease the crisis.

Nonetheless, Lilongwe was quiet that day, and we decided to tarry in search of provisions to take back to the academy. This was a largely thankless venture, but one or two Indian traders had reopened, and we managed to buy some tinned goods. That evening the curfew was lifted, and we learned that one establishment only would be open for business: Pirates' Casino. We drove around the deserted streets, shrouded in darkness because of the ongoing power cut. The casino alone twinkled with light and hummed with the sound of diesel generators.

Several guards sat at the compound gate and beckoned us in to an unexpectedly full car park. Inside, the casino was minimally lit but packed with patrons. Round the edges of the gaming floor, Big Men slumped on sofas, addled with drink; their women nestled close, custodians of the half-drunk bottles of Johnnie Walker set before them. Others from their entourages sat on the floor. I guessed these were Bingu's men, here to flee from the crisis and blot out their cares.

The air was pungent and hazy with sweat and tobacco smoke. We played a little blackjack and made some small wins. As we cashed in our chips, someone peeled off from his master's party and asked us for a Fanta. It was, I think, a roundabout way of offering to indenture himself.

We set off the next day on the long journey through the central plains back to the academy. It took us through a trading centre where I was able to point out a small grocery store, aptly named the 'Money Comes Money Goes Investment Agency'. The roads were still empty, and we made it back in a few hours. There was by now no electricity, running water or phone signal at the academy, but peace reigned, and Dr Highbrow welcomed us in high spirits. He was having coffee and a cigar on his *khonde*, reading Vergil's *Eclogues*.

'*Hic tamen hanc mecum poteras requiescere noctem* – tonight you can rest here with me. The freezer contents are all spoiled. The beef filet is a great loss. But we have the bottled clams of Italy and the garlic and tomatoes of

Mtunthama. I contemplate *spaghetti alle vongole*, if that might tempt you? Duncan has several braziers on the go. "Even now the chimneys are smoking, and the shadows fall longer and longer from the mountain heights . . ."'

The meal was very welcome, and complemented by South African Viognier that we drank from Dr Highbrow's lead crystal glasses. These were an obsession of his which I had noticed early on in our acquaintance. I had invited him to lunch during my first term, and he had asked me in advance if I had 'adequate glassware'. I assured him that I did, but he was clearly disappointed with what I had to offer. He said nothing at the time, but, just before his next visit, he sent over a servant bearing a box of glasses that were to be used instead of my own. It was absurd affectation, but I later came to recognise a noble aspect to the behaviour as well. Fly-by-nighters like myself could treat a few years in Malaŵi as a glorious extended camping trip and have fun 'roughing it'. Insistence on certain high standards of living was Dr Highbrow's declaration of commitment to the country and expressed his contempt for the view that you should cut corners and compromise just because you were in Africa.

Dr Highbrow was much preoccupied with one of his ethnographical projects, and he spoke chiefly of this over dinner, seemingly indifferent to the turmoil spreading through the country. Only afterwards, with whisky by the fire, did he turn to local politics, and then rather philosophically:

'Bingu turns out to be redder in tooth and claw than I had expected – but that may not be wholly to his discredit. His rivals are no less wicked, just more cunning and presentable. Perhaps there is something to be said for a world in which good and evil are luminously opposed, rather than blurred into shades of grey. The contrast can be instructive, even salutary. At least it stimulates outrage and resistance – as you now see.'

His view was at least partly vindicated. A few months later, amid chaos, hyperinflation and pressure from all sides, Bingu suffered a fatal heart attack. It was reported that he had been flown to South Africa for treatment, as Malawîan hospitals were still crippled by shortages of drugs and electricity. Scurrilous rumours abounded, including that he had expired during vigorous intercourse with his second wife.

After a disorderly inter-regnum, Bingu was replaced by Joyce Banda, with great fanfare in the international community, and talk of women leading a political renaissance across the continent. She promised to address all the usual priorities of Western donors, and foreign aid was eagerly funnelled back into the country. Yet she was soon embroiled in Malawî's biggest embezzlement scandal to date. As suitcases of dollars were discovered in the back of cars and under ministers' beds, and an anti-corruption investigator was shot dead at the gates of his own home, the scandal was dubbed 'Cashgate' by the Malawîan press. After two years in office, Joyce Banda was deposed and sent into exile, charged with being the mastermind behind the enormous heist. She embarked on a new career, lecture-touring at distinguished British and American universities, who lionised her as a champion of female empowerment in Africa.

Her successor was Bingu's younger brother, Peter, who immortalised his sibling's memory with a large bronze statue in the capital. 'In pursuing our dreams, not even the sky is the limit,' Bingu was quoted at its unveiling. Peter claimed victory in the so-called 'Tipp-Ex elections' of 2019 but – in an unexpected and stirring development – the result was successfully overturned by the judges of Malawî's Supreme

Court. And so, at the time of writing, Kamuzu Banda's Malaŵi Congress Party has been returned to power for the first time since his downfall, now under the leadership of evangelical pastor Lazarus Chakwera.

XXXIV

THE FORCES OF ENTROPY

'Power all day every day' was the motto of ESCOM, the Electricity Supply Corporation of Malaŵi, when I first arrived in the country. By the time I left, it had been reformulated as '*Towards* power all day every day', but many objected that even this grossly overstated the case. Visitors were often astonished at the dilapidation of Malaŵi's infrastructure: surely things must improve, slowly? they would ask. The answer that they might be getting worse was often met with incredulity, even hostility.

When I occupied my first house, I complained repeatedly about the inadequacy of the water supply. After a few months I persuaded some of the maintenance staff to accompany me in walking the course of the pipes laid beneath the ground. We trudged through dry scrub forest but, after about a mile, came to a blooming oasis, with mature palm trees springing from rich, moist ground. We had identified the leak: it must have been there for years.

Malaŵian entropy, Dr Highbrow called it: the process by which everything – buildings, roads, vehicles, government agencies, volunteer projects, kitchen utensils, universal joints – seemed to fall apart faster or at least more obviously than anywhere else. The forces of destruction operated voraciously before your very eyes, a reminder of how much unseen energy is required just to keep up the fabric of civilisation.

No doubt Africa only exaggerated processes that were also active in the West. I sensed that we failed to notice the same decay back at home because our inheritance was so vast it seemed imperishable. The erosion of a cathedral becomes apparent only over decades; a mud hut might be washed away in a single monsoon.

The default position, I came to believe, was that of the peasant farmers, who eked out a bare existence from the unyielding earth. That was remarkable enough, and anything more demanded a miracle of human achievement.

A few miles from Kamuzu Academy lies Wimbe, a trading centre made famous by William Kamkwamba and his memoir, *The Boy Who Harnessed the Wind*. I regularly passed through Wimbe on my way to Lysard Moyo and the tobacco farm. It is a wretched place, far from any paved road, with most buildings in disrepair, many just empty shells. Everything has a blasted appearance recalling news footage of war-torn places, though Wimbe has in fact known at least a hundred years of peace.

The town's one, broad street has a row of single-storey concrete buildings on either side, wilderness beyond. The dirt road turns into deep quagmire during the rains, and I remember one day sheltering from a downpour under the eaves of a shop, watching the town attempt to conduct its business. In the middle of the road, a van was stuck deep in a river of mud, from which another vehicle was failing to tow it. I could smell the fumes from the futile revving of the diesel engines. Nearby, a young mother was trying to cross the road with an infant on her back, and another child struggling beside her. They were knee deep in brown water and had to wrest their feet free of the sludgy sediment with every step. It was like the landscapes in

World War One photographs of Passchendaele. Another vehicle skidded around her, not wanting to slow down for fear of losing momentum and also getting stuck. Beside me, a throng of young men were loitering outside the boozing parlour, grumbling because a power cut had put an end to their music.

It was here, improbably enough, that Kamkwamba lived and 'harnessed the wind'. The main action of his memoir takes place in the early 2000s, during the drought and famine that occurred under the government of Banda's successor, Muluzi. As the population of Wimbe starved to death before his eyes, Kamkwamba became fascinated by electricity and constructed a windmill from refuse. He attached this to a dynamo, which then powered a water pump. The irrigation was intended to allow a second annual growing season, so that his family would no longer be wholly dependent on erratic seasonal rains.

Kamkwamba's deeply moving story reveals much about Malaŵi at that period. There is a strong suggestion of the societal breakdown that followed the end of Banda's rule, with painful anecdotes of how village kinsmen exploited each other's desperation and of how the power of the chiefs to unite their people was undermined. In one painful episode, Chief Wimbe is beaten by Muluzi's thugs for speaking out against the government, and faith in his authority is shattered forever.

Kamkwamba's uniqueness is the most arresting feature of the book. Indeed, one obstacle he faced – omitted from the film adaptation – is that his ingenuity was so extraordinary as to attract accusations of witchcraft from his fellow villagers. But when word of his achievement spread beyond Wimbe, Kamkwamba was feted as a hero, and won sponsorship to leave Malaŵi and study abroad. Through his book he achieved celebrity in the West and, by the time I arrived at the academy, he was in America giving TED talks on development. That was a decade after his original project, yet – to judge from the appearance of Wimbe – Kamkwamba might never have existed. As one local aid worker incisively put it: 'Why hasn't anyone else harnessed the wind?'

We like to imagine that every problem in the world has its technical solution, if only it can be identified and implemented. But the reality of Wimbe confounded this view, suggesting instead only the wild improbability of progress. To erect a single windmill required a lightning bolt of originality to strike in the right place, but to raise an entire society needed numberless miracles of this sort to be repeated in close proximity over decades or centuries. And any advance quickly evanesced without vigorous pro-activity to maintain it.

From Banda's palace at Nguru-ya-Nawambe, you drive west to Kasungu National Park, passing the remains of the once international airport built primarily to connect that residence with the outside world. Unused since the fall of the regime, the short runway is now scarred and overgrown, the waiting room an empty shell. Two abandoned aircraft boarding stairs form eerie dinosauric silhouettes against the flat, unbroken horizon.

Driving past this, the villages become fewer and the vegetation denser until you reach the park and are enclosed in thick, level forest. It is, in the words of Flemings, 'a fierce place'. Poachers are many and animals few. The elephants, hippos and lions that remain are shy and retiring until disturbed, whereupon they can become very aggressive. 'This is not the Kruger Park,' I was warned. 'If you see animals at Kasungu, you are probably too close to them.' Nevertheless, the place has an exceptional calm, especially at dawn, when the fish eagles swoop over the reservoir and warthogs prance about in the morning coolness. Its endless brachystegia woodland is a uniform blend of brown, silver, yellow and green which confers, all year round, the hues and atmosphere of early autumn in Europe. The gates of the park were about forty miles from the academy, and I visited frequently, often enjoying the place to myself. Tourists were few, and the last remaining lodge had been recently deserted after its German proprietor got trampled to death by an elephant in the course of a Boxing Day stroll.

Dr Highbrow and I became acquainted with the park's wildlife scouts, who one day showed us some of its more unexpected treasures. At the headquarters, a massive steel door was pushed open to reveal a magazine, in which heaps of drab unpolished ivory and battered sable horns were piled. M16s, Lee–Enfields, poachers' homemade flintlocks and huge calibre elephant guns lay casually discarded on the floor in various conditions of disrepair. Clumsily opened, half-empty ammunition boxes were stacked in towers that swayed precariously as you stepped past.

'Do you ever use any of these?' I asked.

Our scout nodded with enthusiasm. Yes, only last month, he explained, they had tracked a party of poachers for days through the forest. After the poachers killed an elephant, the scout and his men concealed themselves in thickets around the carcass. The next morning, when the poachers returned to carve up the meat and excise the tusks, the scouts unleashed their ambush. He picked up one of the M16s and brandished it excitedly: that was the very weapon he had used. They had shot all the men dead and tipped their bodies into a dry gully.

Next we visited the scientific research station. Its tin roof was falling in, the window panes all gone, the interior jammed with broken furniture. Animal specimens floated in jars, chaotically dispersed on shelves and in cupboards. Inspecting them more closely, I noticed that most bore labels identifying the collector, date and specimen by its Latin and common names. It was clear that, for many years, these had been collected fastidiously, labelled with brown ink in neat copperplate handwriting. With the passage of time, however, the specimens grew fewer, the labels more and more careless. Then I found the last, in a jar with a shred of paper taped ineptly to its side. In a non-cursive biro script had been scrawled the single word 'snake'.

Drawers and cupboards produced mephitic dust-clouds from the crumbling of desiccated birds and rodents. Horns and pelts, hides and feathers were stuffed into boxes; a crocodile skin mouldered under a desk. Two vast cabinets contained slender drawers, all precisely labelled with index cards in brass mountings: 'Grasses A–C', 'Grasses D–F' and so on.

I thought of the episode in Conrad's *Heart of Darkness* when the protagonist Marlow chances upon a solitary abandoned shack in the course of his river journey through the desolation of the Belgian Congo. Inside, he finds a tattered volume entitled *An Inquiry into Some Points of Seamanship*. 'Not a very enthralling book,' he observes. 'But at first glance you could see there a singleness of intention, an honest concern for the right way of going to work, which made these humble pages [. . .] luminous with another than a professional light.'

The stolid little book Marlow finds offers an antidote to the chaos and destruction all around him, and I felt the same way about those trays of grasses. It was not the contents that were important but the order and discipline they represented. As a foil to brutality and neglect, that humdrum work appeared humane, even illustrious. There was no technical formula to arrest decay, let alone guarantee progress. But the examples of Wimbe, Kamkwamba and that research station hinted at the existence of a moral bedrock more important than any material structure built upon it.

XXXV

THE AGONY IN THE GARDEN

Time and again, the world of the village survived disaster, so that it sometimes seemed far more robust than my own. On the surface, the turmoil wrought by Bingu, for example, barely caused a ripple. The peasant farmers did not want for fuel or forex, as they had never possessed either. What mattered to them was rain, which Bingu could neither give nor take. In fact, the influence of government, for good or ill, felt very faint away from the capital.

Still, there was an interface between the village and the outside world, and it was at this point that calamity could strike most cruelly. Modern healthcare, though far from universally available, was provided just widely enough that its absence could be felt, often painfully. Within weeks of the forex crisis, shortages of HIV drugs began to be experienced, aggravated by theft and black-marketeering. Those unlucky enough to need inpatient treatment found their hospitals in even worse conditions than usual.

I had befriended Moses Mkango, the senior clinical officer at Saint Luke's, a nearby hospital. I was by then due to return to England to study medicine as a second degree, and I wanted to observe his work. He and his wife were both employed at the hospital, and their family lived in one of the better houses in Mtunthama: a sturdy bungalow from the Kamuzu Banda period, painted blue and yellow, with ferns and creepers growing about the *khonde*.

Saint Luke's was large for a rural hospital, and relatively well endowed by churches and overseas charities. It had an operating theatre, maternity unit, half a dozen wards and various outpatient clinics. But, as in many Malaŵian hospitals, there were no doctors, only clinical officers. These are the backbone of the country's healthcare system, though they are trained for just two years before being dispatched to the provinces, expected to crack on with whatever comes through the door: complex medical patients, major surgery, difficult deliveries, polytrauma, dying children.

You never forget your first experience of a rural hospital in Malaŵi. It is dark, dirty, and it smells. The wards are crowded, with patients sharing beds or sleeping on a floor grimy with dust, dressings and discarded medical equipment. Relatives throng around, on or under every bed. They do much of the nursing, prepare food at the bedside, attempt to shoo away the gathering flies. Hundreds of pairs of eyes fixate on your entry, then follow you expectantly. At first you have just a general impression of suffering humanity concentrated in one space. It takes a while to notice the details, but, as your eyes adjust, you spot advanced pathology everywhere.

Even before Bingu's crisis really struck, Moses had already gone several months without wages. The provision of salaries to public servants was commonly disrupted, and he had continued to work unpaid, subsisting on the labour of tenants who farmed his small plot of land. Things became harder as the shortages began to bite. At the height of the catastrophe, Moses found himself running a hospital that increasingly lacked even the most basic drugs and equipment. Many patients he had to just turn away; others needed to be operated on urgently. He was doing emergency surgery, obstetric and orthopaedic procedures without painkillers or anaesthetics. He told me how his patients had to be held down, in the manner of eighteenth-century barber-surgeons.

Stolidly, indomitably, with patience and even good humour, Moses just got on with his work. He was not much inclined to comment on the situation, but at length I pressed him for an opinion. When he answered, I thought I could detect the smallest flicker of a smile at his mouth's edge: 'The discipline of political science would appear not to be flourishing in Malaŵi at present.'

If I fell seriously ill, I could hope to get out of the country if it became necessary, though just thinking about that challenge was unsettling. But all those who could not even dream of treatment elsewhere seemed unperturbed by the unfolding catastrophe. I suppose many were so unaccustomed to having any healthcare at all that the lack of it now seemed of less importance.

Conditions were bad, even at the best of times. When I first accompanied Moses on one of his ward rounds, he saw a man in his forties who had pneumonia, TB, HIV and malaria. He was dying, but Moses decided to give him a try in the hospital's 'intensive care unit' – the one ward that had its own nurse, and provision to supply nasal oxygen to a single patient. At least a dozen relatives had settled themselves on the floor around the patient's bed in wide-eyed silence. They were packed so densely that Moses could not reach over them to connect the oxygen concentrator to the wall socket. He therefore handed the plug to one of the relatives and beckoned him to insert it into the mains. The young man looked embarrassedly from plug to socket and back again. He had absolutely no idea what to do with it. Moses stretched to plug it in himself, and everyone watched intently, in expectation of wondrous results. Nothing happened – there was another power cut.

Moses' ward rounds left a brief wake of order, soon lost in the sea of chaos. Blood transfusions were rare and mostly depended on a lucky match with a donor relative. Mismatch was common, and I observed Moses attend a young woman with malaria as she suffered a severe transfusion reaction. She was struggling to breathe, and her eyes were wild with terror, but Moses calmly stopped the blood and managed to stabilise her. She began to recover well.

The next day, he found her bed empty and asked if she had been discharged. One of the nurses sheepishly explained that she had not. In fact, she had been restarted overnight on the same transfusion, sustained the same reaction, and this time she had died. There were no recriminations. It was seen as a routine consequence of the disarray that prevailed in such an understaffed, ill-equipped hospital. The relatives thanked everyone for doing their best and left to go about their mourning.

Just outside, an elderly hospital gardener was tending an elaborate flowering border of hibiscus and bougainvillea, set among neatly trimmed hedging. The soil was freshly turned and meticulously weeded. I was surveying it with a Scottish doctor who was also visiting the hospital. Beyond the planted area, broken steps led up to the cracked concrete walkway, under the subsiding roof, to the missing doors of the main entrance. On either side, you could peer through broken windows into the unillumined wards.

'Typical that they put all that effort into the garden when nothing else is working,' my companion observed. 'Why couldn't they spend the money on something useful?'

It was a compelling argument from a utilitarian point of view, but I had to disagree. The garden probably cost almost nothing to maintain – but even that wasn't really the point. The gardener was setting an example for all to see, of doing his job, and doing it well. He presented a humble vision of order, beauty, even hope. Had I been entering the hospital as a patient, it might have been the only thing there that reassured me.

XXXVI

LUX IN TENEBRIS

Gratitude and forbearance were conspicuous in every patient I met at Saint Luke's. An elderly epileptic had multiple chronic wounds from burns sustained by falling into fires while convulsing. I remembered reading how epileptics were, in other countries on the continent, even known as 'the burned' for precisely this reason. Every week, this man shambled two miles on his swollen, purulent legs to have them cleaned and re dressed. The bandages by then would be heavily soiled with dust and exudate, the wounds hideous, painful and malodorous.

He spoke good English and told me his family were fearful of his seizures. His wife was in fact too scared to live with him, he explained without reproach. She and her family still did most of his cooking, and for that he was thankful, as most of his burns were from cooking fires. But now it was winter, he felt the cold and sometimes slept by a fire for warmth. This had been the source of his most recent injury.

He had once been some kind of clerk in local government before falling on hard times. Out of respect for the hospital, he put on a threadbare suit and tie whenever he attended. There was, when he spoke, not a trace of bitterness or self-pity. He was cheerful, warm, thankful and intelligent. He winced with pain and then laughed as the bandages were peeled from his angry, fragile skin. He smiled indomitably through tears that welled up to make his eyes still brighter. The clinical officer coated the sores with a thick layer of granulated sugar before applying fresh bandages. It worked as an antibacterial agent in the absence of anything better. When they were done, he beamed with thanks and contentment, delightedly stroking the clean, neat dressings. Still smiling, he took up his stick and hobbled back home to resume his hardships.

I never ceased to be astonished by the resilience of these patients. There was a capacity to endure physical pain that I would never have believed possible: I saw open fractures manipulated and painful gynaecological procedures done without anaesthetics. (Did the women have an even higher pain threshold than the men?) And there was this immense mental stoicism that confronted suffering with cheerfulness and optimism.

'God is great!' was Mussa's only comment as he stared at his bleeding forearm, which the broken electric metal saw had flayed down to the bone. He had been working under my car, with the tool's leads stretched into my kitchen, and two exposed wires jammed roughly into the plug socket. The aged blade had snapped and then flown off with force, and Mussa's instant reaction was to give thanks – I presumed for not having lost his hand. I had to restrain my dog from licking up the fragments of flesh and droplets of blood which the blade had scattered about the lawn. 'God is great,' Mussa repeated solemnly. The engine of the car was being substantially deconstructed, and there was no one else to take him, so Mussa got on his bike and cycled the couple of miles to the hospital, clutching the bleeding wound.

Confronted by injury and illness, exigency and acts of God, village Malaŵians seemed able to withstand anything, and I came to admire them as an almost invincible people. However, when I later returned to Malaŵi to work at an urban hospital surrounded by slums, what I saw was different. There the suffering seemed all too often wrought by man, and the result was abjection.

Everyone suffered, but the women seemed to have it worst: violence, rape and HIV made for a common and terrible combination. Many of the girls were without family or worked as prostitutes. I came to recognise an almost dead expression as they were told, often rather casually, that they were infected with the virus. It struck me how blankly, silently, acceptingly they received the news, as if ruination had already been inflicted long before.

One young teenager, my colleagues established, was an orphan who had inherited her mother's tiny home brewery in one of the city's roughest quarters. She had been exploited by other residents after her mother's death: they told her they would only buy her beer if they could also have sex with her. She had been doing that for over a year, and had now been admitted with HIV and an associated opportunistic infection. In her glassy eyes and muted answers, I sensed an apathy, as though her mind had shut down because unable to compute further anguish. All that remained was a body which might suddenly awaken to physical pain – as when the clinician had to perform a lumbar puncture on her without anaesthetic.

On the other hand, I remember also a village girl, with mild learning difficulties, who lived on a tobacco estate near the academy. One day she was raped in a field as she walked home by a young man she knew. The local community turned on him, and he was beaten by a mob armed with sticks. A week later, I saw the girl going about her day, superficially cheerful. The crime and her suffering were no less real, but it was a world apart from the mental desolation that seemed so obvious in the victims from the city. A tight little community had fallen in immediately behind the village girl to offer justice, protection and comfort. The absence of any of these in the urban slums presumably allowed the most pernicious crime to flourish without hindrance or mitigation.

Such experiences sometimes made me recoil from Malaŵian life in horror, but it was essential to maintain a sense of perspective. My work in UK hospitals has long since alerted me to our own society's capacity for nastiness, though we certainly sweep it aside better. I once expected the cruelty inflicted on the young beer seller to be the worst I would ever encounter, but then I visited a prison in the UK, and met some of its psychiatrist's patients. Three had been gang-raped on British council estates, one so violently that her ear had been bitten off in the process. Africa has no monopoly on horror; in fact, just as Conrad meant to suggest to his European readers, its real source might actually be closer to home.

But suffering in Malaŵi was more widespread, and often seemed unmitigated by reflexes, personal and institutional, which we take for granted in the West. Indeed, you might find cruelty precisely where you would hope for compassion. In another Malaŵian urban hospital, I encountered a young man who had been transferred from the nearby prison. He was not my patient, but for some reason I was stirred to approach him. He was set apart from the rest in a dingy corner of the ward, and there was something indefinably wrong about his presence there. A policeman sat beside him in the gloom, eating his lunch and playing a game on his phone.

As I approached, I saw that the man's legs and one arm were handcuffed to the metal bed frame. I could not establish why he was a prisoner, but I learned he was a paraplegic, rumoured to have broken his back long before. There was a terrible smell in the air and I lifted the blankets. Underneath he was caked in weeks of his own ordure. He had numerous deep bed sores, prominently exposed to the bone. Several were thickly smeared with mixed dry and wet excrement, and maggots writhed among them.

I put back the blankets and just kept myself from vomiting. The man then whimpered and opened his eyes. He was delirious, but the terror in his face was unmistakable. I approached the nurses and asked if they knew about him. They just muttered something about him being a prisoner, so I went back to re-expose the blankets. Then they too recoiled in horror and would not come any closer. There was nothing they could do while he was chained to the bed, one explained. I asked about the handcuffs. The guard didn't have the key. I was now causing a small disturbance. He had smiled at me indulgently at first, but now he stood up and ushered me from the room.

I asked questions, found a supposedly responsible clinician, bothered people, tried to get the man moved elsewhere, but it was useless. He died of sepsis the same afternoon. I was told he had been cleaned up and accorded some measure of dignity, but I did not feel particularly convinced by these assurances. I sensed that my enquiry was being discouraged.

I slept badly that night but better the night after, and then my life went on as before. Even so, I have often thought about that man and his mistreatment, which resulted less from malevolence than from indifference: of the prison and medical staff to his worsening condition; of the guard as he ate lunch while his charge rotted in agony before him. The indifference of the nurses as they shrugged their shoulders in helplessness. My own indifference when I balked at creating trouble, making a scene, getting my own hands dirty. When I slept soundly after just one unsettled night. To put ourselves in another's shoes is our constant, elusive challenge. How little my own experience and imagination could teach me of what he had gone through.

As I witnessed more of the immense suffering taking place in the background of Malaŵian life, I might have distanced myself from the pontifications of Dr Highbrow. While men died horribly, he was holding forth about Latin and Greek literature, to inattentive pupils, in a perverse dictator's fantasy school: what could be more painfully absurd? But the Malaŵian experience is topsy-turvy, and that was not what I felt. Quite the opposite: Dr Highbrow's lessons suddenly seemed vitally important.

Here he is teaching Vergil to his GCSE set. Aeneas has escaped the carnage of the Trojan War and is wandering around the Mediterranean with his people. In their search for a new homeland, they arrive at a strange city. They are weary, destitute and fearful of this unfamiliar place. I wondered how many of Dr Highbrow's pupils, scooped from distant villages into the strange world of Kamuzu Academy, had experienced similar feelings themselves.

Before encountering anyone, Aeneas and his men chance upon a fresco, outside on the city wall. With relief they see that it depicts the horrors of war with obvious pity. *sunt lacrimae rerum et mentem mortalia tangunt* – 'They shed tears for these things,' Aeneas concludes about the city's residents. 'Mortal things touch their hearts.' It is a moment of relief and exaltation, as Aeneas realises these people must be alive to human suffering if they think it worth exploring in their art. He can appeal to them for sympathy.

Or perhaps Dr Highbrow is discussing the *Iliad* with his sixth form. In the epic's final scene, after years of unbridled violence, iron-hearted Achilles for once feels pity. Imagining his enemy's grief, he hands over the body of Hector, Priam's dead son, for which the father has come begging. It is a brief truce only, a flash in the darkness, and the war is presently resumed. But that fleeting, improbable moment of kindness and understanding is preserved for us in Homer – if only we would pass it on.

These are moments of epiphany, miracles of sensitivity within the context of our everyday indifference. They have been recorded and transmitted across millennia, through art, literature, religion and ceremony. They form the store of human sympathy from which all our civilised reflexes derive; however, these are delicate and require cultivation. If we fail in this, we revert to a state of moral exigency, in which suffering leaves us staring blankly into our phones, or running feebly from the darkness.

XXXVII

LAND OF FIRE

'Land of fire' is the usual gloss on 'Malaŵi', the name chosen by Banda at independence. The etymology is uncertain: it derives from an ancient kingdom – Maravi – which ruled the area, but the word also seems to have meant 'flames'. Why the land should have had this association is unclear. Was it suggested by the peculiar play of light when its lake glows at dawn? Or rather by the prevalence of brick-burning and iron-smelting in the period before the arrival of Europeans? Or did it refer to the centrality of fire in the country's creation myths?

Though the written word came only recently to Malaŵi, the country's tribes have many myths, orally transmitted, like the early epics of Greece. The most profound explain the creation of man and the necessity of death. According to the Chewa, Chiuta – God – created people and animals together, and then dwelled among them. All lived harmoniously on earth, enjoying immortality and plenty, until man discovered fire and destroyed paradise. The animals fled from the burning forests, and Chiuta left to make a new home for himself in heaven, where he invented rain. He quenched the blaze and saved the world from annihilation, but, at the same time, he invented death. He rescinded man's immortality so he could take the departed souls up to heaven, there to labour at the production of rain. And so the world assumed its cycle: humans create fire on earth, and the rising smoke alerts the ancestors above, stirring them to douse the flames.

The story explains the origin of death – but also its unreality. Afterlife is assured: the spirits of the departed merely pass to 'the village on the other side'. There the ancestors continue to serve and guide the living and the unborn, and the contact between the two worlds is sustained by reverence and propitiation.

This story, first transcribed by missionaries and ethnographers, became the major source of inspiration for Malaŵi's poets and playwrights, with all addressing it somewhere in their work. A few took it as their major theme, reimagining and reconfiguring the myth to the point of obsession. Poet Innocent Banda presented his version as a calligram: 'Man the Inventor', is reproduced at the end of this chapter.

The more time I spent in Malaŵi, the more I thought I could discern the images and precepts of the myth in thinking and behaviour across the land. Innocent Banda's poem evoked the deep conservatism of the Malaŵian village, which seemed an echo of the ancestors' dismay at man's first Promethean experiment. The myth also proclaimed that death shall have no dominion, in accord with the courage and resilience so widely observable. The material world had been conceived as a divine gift: did this go some way to explaining the gratitude that so often defied privation? In the appetite for Christian worship, I sensed a harmony with the myth's insistence on original sin, while *gule wamkulu* expressed an impulse to revert to prelapsarian animal innocence. 'Is there any hope of reconciliation between man and Chiuta? Man and animal?' asked Steve Chimombo, perhaps Malaŵi's greatest reinventor of ancient legend in his play 'The Rainmaker':

Haven't I with my own eyes
seen the eternal circles
rejoin and reconcile?

I saw man dancing with animal
animal dancing with spirit
spirit dancing with man

Animal, man, spirit
dancing the Great Dance
of the world.

Gule wamkulu had once been called *pemphero lalikulu* – not the Great Dance, but the Great Prayer. It was a ritual of atonement for man's transgressions against the animal world and God. As in the myth, atonement was needed to summon rain.

Rain, a matter of universal, existential importance, had fire as its counterpart. Every year, at the start of the planting season, Malaŵi's landscape smoulders with offerings burnt to appease the ancestors. As the smoke rises to heaven, rain should fall to earth, it was explained to me – a process of sympathetic magic. In times of drought, rain prayers would be ordained by tribal chiefs and village headmen, by members of parliament and the president himself. They were offered in churches, mosques and in myriad pagan ceremonies. Near the academy, Dr Highbrow had witnessed rain invoked by animal sacrifice, the detail of the rites exactly as described by Jack Mapanje in 'Before Chilembwe Tree':

> Now, here I seat my gourd of beer,
> On my little fire, throw my millet
> Flour and my smoked meat [. . .]

> The goat blood on the rock
> The smoke that issued
> The drums you danced to
> And the rains hoped for—

Kamuzu Banda was admired for his power as a rainmaker. Sangala told the story of how his father had once walked out into parched fields, there to hold aloft the village radio, as Kamuzu's voice was broadcast from Sanjika Palace in Blantyre. Even from that enormous distance, Sangala explained, the voice could command the heavens and – lo! – there fell rain.

The weather was a particular focus of interest for witches. I first arrived at Kamuzu Academy in a period of drought, and it was no coincidence that there occurred at the same time a spate of witch aeroplane crashes. I saw none of these myself, but they were described to me vividly by Flemings and Sangala.

The first had taken place in broad daylight on market day, in the middle of Mtunthama. Everyone had been astonished to see the witch glide past very low, almost at head height, and then crash into a tree. The whole market fell upon him with their fists. But what was most astonishing, Sangala related, was that when this man was apprehended, they found that, instead of a nose, he had a long yellow beak, like a bird. He was quickly identified as the cause of the drought, and the villagers beat him soundly and drove him away.

Had a witch ever been killed in these parts? I asked.

Yes – once – a few years before, Sangala answered. A young girl had died of apparently natural causes, but the father found out that she had in fact been poisoned by a witch, whom he then murdered.

'Did he get into trouble?'

'No. He was very quick. He struck quickly – with his knife – so the witch had no time to put a curse on him.'

'I meant with the police – did he get arrested for the murder?'

'Ah no, there was no problem. Because the police – they also knew that man was a witch.'

When I last revisited Malaŵi, there was talk of a disturbance that had occurred a few weeks earlier, just outside the academy gates. It all started with the death of a young man, noteworthy because his father was a local chief and also a gardener at the school. The chief's other son had gone to the cemetery to prepare the grave, but when he got there he found a laptop bag hanging from the branch of a tree. Inside was out-of-date paper money and a charm.

Charms are witches' utensils: small, nasty-looking objects made of beads and twigs, gourds and thorns, fastened together with feathers and twine. There were excellent examples in the museum in Blantyre, each set beside an explanatory note. 'This charm can make you invisible,' read one; 'This charm will make you rich,' another. 'This charm is to kill your enemies.'

The man took the charm back to his village to consult the elders. There, before their very eyes, it turned itself into a cat, which began mocking them. Realising they were threatened by black magic, they tried to kill the animal but somehow were prevented from doing so. They were clearly out of their depth, so took the whole story – and the cat – to the local policeman, who occupies a lonely booth on the nearest tarmac road.

The long arm of the law acted decisively: he led them all to the large ornamental roundabout outside the academy and there, before a crowd of tense onlookers, doused laptop bag, money and cat with petrol, and set everything alight.

As the smoke rose, it was again explained to me, rain began to fall.

'But, Mr Sangala,' I asked, 'who left the bag at the graveyard?'

'The witch,' he answered surely.

'Which witch?'

'The cat.'

'The witch turned himself into a cat?'

'Yes! The same witch stopping the rain for many weeks!'

'Why should the witch want to stop the rain?'

Sangala thought about this for a time and then admitted he was not sure.

'Sometimes witches are going on a long journey, and they do not want to walk in the mud,' he suggested uncertainly. 'Also, sometimes a witch is burning bricks, so he does not want the rain to stop his brick-making.'

'Fair enough,' I answered.

Sangala then paused again before adding: 'Also, some witches – they just don't like the rain!'

'You seem to know a lot about witches, Mr Sangala,' I ventured.

He gave me an enigmatic smile. 'Some people, they even think I am a witch!' He then looked serious: 'I am not a witch. But if you want, I can take you to see – *the things of the witches*. I can take you to meet a witch. And if you want, he can even change *you* into a witch.'

'Is that a good idea?'

'It depends.'

'Depends on what?'

'On whether you want to know what it is to be a witch!'

'Would it be dangerous?'

'Only if you use your magic to hurt someone. If you hurt someone with your magic, and their magic is stronger, then your magic will come back against you instead.'

'Well, I don't want to hurt anyone, Mr Sangala. But I don't think I want to become a witch. I mean, could I change back?'

'Oh yes, of course,' he answered straightforwardly. 'Becoming a witch is like putting on a shirt. When you want to stop being a witch, you take off the shirt.'

I considered but did not take up Sangala's offer. I thought of Racey and the rain shrines, and decided some things should only be looked into so far. But the episode suggested ingrained reflexes that again tallied with the ancient myths. They might manifest as baleful superstition: even as I write, I learn from the Malaŵian online news of a man recently stoned to death because suspected of wizardry, and of a woman sawn in half for witchcraft. But the source of such behaviour was deep and mysterious. Who was I to say it did not also supply some of the vast inner strength that enabled these people to endure?

MAN THE INVENTOR

            A
         cloud
            rose
               from the East
                  the North
                     and West
                  smoke rose—
               for Chiuta
               fled
                  to the sky.
                     It was a flame
                     that caused
                     the smoke
                     and set
                     the world
                     a-spinning
                       on the path
                       to destruction.
                          Intellect's a load
                       too heavy on man
                          flames destroy
                       man's home
                  flames await
Man, concealed in innocent looking metals.
            It was a moth I laughed at
               last night; that
                  from the dark
                     discovers
                        a light
               and in jubilation burns itself.

XXXVIII

SIGNIFICANT SOIL

At another Malaŵian hospital I met Hans, an elderly surgeon from Europe who had lived briefly in the country decades before and then returned in retirement to work as a volunteer. Malaŵi and surgery were the passions of his life, and he had resolved to consecrate his remaining years to their service.

I was fortunate to assist him with one of his operating lists, and its scope and variety were extraordinary. He was a gastro-intestinal surgeon by training, but that day moved between bowel and bladder, neuro- and cardiothoracic surgery. He took a hand-drill to a boy's skull to relieve blood on the brain, fixed a gynaecological procedure that had gone badly wrong and excised a sinister-looking tumour the size of a grapefruit from a young man's chest wall. With a couple of ribs removed, I was able to peer at a human heart beating inside the body.

Hans's proudest achievement was his burns unit. He had found a plastic surgeon friend back at home, and assisted him with some skin grafts. He then whipped up funds to buy the necessary equipment, which he brought back to Malaŵi.

I watched him take what looked like a tiny carpentry plane and glide it over the anaesthetised child's thigh. It sliced off a neat, rectangular sliver of skin, leaving behind a shallow patch of exposed fatty tissue, which quickly turned from white to pink as the shaved capillaries began to bleed. This wound was then dressed as the surgeon turned his attention to the piece of skin he had harvested. It was placed inside the dermatome, which resembled a tiny mangle, manufactured in dull grey metal to a level of superb precision. The bladed rollers were turned, and the patch of skin scored with a tight criss-cross pattern. When this was removed, you could just see the incisions, but it looked otherwise the same.

Then came the magic: with this patch of skin floated in a dish of saline, he stretched it out with forceps and the whole thing was transformed into a broad lattice or net, exquisitely fine, and many times its original surface area. This was spread over the gaping burn on the child's torso, tethered in place, and then dressed. Hans inspected the graft over the next few days and murmured his contentment as the lattice pattern became blurry at the edges, with tiny margins of new skin beginning to grow.

Burns were common, especially among children. This was the result of food preparation taking place almost universally on open cooking fires of wood or charcoal, in tiny huts, using broken utensils and clumsy battered pots without lids or handles.

Most of the victims who came into the unit had hideous burns – anything less severe would scarcely justify the great distances the patients had covered to get there. Many were full thickness and covered extensive areas. The children were in variable states when they came in: a few screamed in agony, others just whimpered or stared blankly, as though so crushed by pain they could no longer express it. Some were shut down and near death on arrival.

The associated ward was like others in Malaŵi: the room was dim, the floor dirty concrete, the beds densely packed and rickety, the air swarming with flies. But over every child was positioned a small, cage-like frame of welded iron. From this blankets could be suspended, to protect the children from cold, dust and insects, without touching their vulnerable flesh. These little cages served an essential function, but, given the context, their resemblance to cooking griddles was unsettling.

It was surprisingly quiet by the standards of other children's wards, as though everyone was just too overwhelmed to cry, but the peace was suddenly shattered by an eruption of violent wailing. This was how a death was customarily signalled by gathered relatives.

In this case, a young girl had come in scorched so badly from neck to feet that she died soon after arrival. At the moment of her passing, there arose a furious lament from the large group of relatives around her bed. Tears fell profusely, with faces so contorted they looked like a cubist's stylised vision of human suffering. As one howling voice fell, another rose in its place, to create a continuous wall of sound. And they made all the same gestures, tearing hair, beating breasts, falling to their knees and pressing faces to the filthy ground. They seemed unitary: less like individuals than a single body and soul, screaming without inhibition. It was strangely vigorous and alive, and could not have contrasted more forcefully with the tiny mutilated body, silent and motionless, around which they wept.

Such strength and solidarity were beyond my comprehension, but Dylan Thomas had seen children burned to death during the Blitz. His response was a challenging poem, 'A Refusal to Mourn the Death, by Fire, of a Child in London':

[. . .] I shall not murder
The mankind of her going with a grave truth
Nor blaspheme down the stations of the breath
With any further
Elegy of innocence and youth.

Deep with the first dead lies London's daughter,
Robed in the long friends,
The grains beyond age, the dark veins of her mother,
Secret by the unmourning water
Of the riding Thames.
After the first death, there is no other.

Like the Chewa mythology, Thomas's poem insisted that death was illusory, merely part of a bigger cosmic process in which you never cease to participate. The friendly worms that consume the girl's body are one with the soil and lifeblood of the mother who bore her. We do not die, only return to the parental embrace of the life-giving earth.

How consoling really is this conception of death? As an individual, it brought me little comfort. But I tried to imagine how it might mean more to a community, who knew they must endure despite one member's passing. The poem speaks of belonging: London's daughter finds her grave beside the Thames, the location twice affirmed, which I had always found odd in a poem that celebrates the universal. But it made sense as I considered the mourning women, who would take their burnt girl home and bury her in their midst, as Lysard Moyo had done with his daughter. She would remain physically present among the living, nourishing and consecrating their soil, affirming their right to dwell there.

According to another Chewa legend, the first man and woman made their home on a hilltop called Kaphirintiwa. Their footsteps and the imprints of their tools were there stamped magically into the rock, connecting their descendants with the site forever. It was said that the marks could still be seen so, one fine spring day, Dr Highbrow and I set off to find them. We knew the hill was somewhere within a forest reserve not far from the capital, occasionally frequented by bird-watchers, but otherwise mostly ignored by tourists. A little groundwork was needed to obtain a guide, but eventually we were introduced to an old man who agreed to take us to the place.

We ambled several hours through woodland thronging with birds and butterflies, crossed gentle brooks and waded through bracken. Then we came upon a kiln for smelting: a giant clay funnel, sunken, cracked and sprouting with foliage and wild flowers. I had seen similar elsewhere in Malaŵi, iron-age relics that were active as late as the 1930s. This one was the only trace of human activity as far as the eye could see.

We hauled ourselves up a steep rocky staircase, clutching at tufts of shrub to steady our ascent. At the summit we gazed east through mists to Banda's city, west over the dark forests of Mozambique. All around, the boundless sky glowed orange with cloud and iridescence after a spell of light rain.

There followed some uncertainty as details from the myth were identified. Here – no! there – was man's first footstep on earth. Our guide pointed to an oblong indentation in the granite. A second smaller one was explained as the first woman's. There was their original maize mortar, a small concave boulder. That forked crack in the rock was the imprint of their hoe. We traipsed on: a shallow pool was the winnowing basket they had used to separate maize from chaff for the first time.

We were skeptical of these attributions but enchanted by the strange atmosphere of the place, with its preternatural stillness and dazzling haze. Our guide could not be persuaded to take us to an associated shrine, which was perhaps evidence that it was still active. But as we ventured to the edge of the peak, we noticed two small and shabby bowls of plastic, filled with maize beer and millet seed sodden with rain. They were votive offerings, mouldy but fairly recently left there. '*Numen inest!*' Dr Highbrow exclaimed – some god is in this place.

The Kaphirintiwa myth implied a point of transition, from nomadic to settled life in one place. The hallmarks of this were crop cultivation, house-building and burial, a triad that still captured perfectly the essence of the Malaŵian village, with its corn fields, brick kiln and coffin workshop. Even the most important tools of its daily life remained identical to those described in the legend.

A boy receives his first hoe in an affirmation of his manhood. It is sometimes the only durable object he will ever possess. The mortar is the woman's symbol of abundance. I remember a *gule* dance in which husband and wife bush pigs cavorted together around a mortar. The wife bush pig then lay on the floor, keeping it clenched between her thighs, while the husband pranced above her, thrusting rhythmically into it with the enormous, phallic pestle. Teeming crowds of children whooped delightedly at this suggestive display, and the maize burst green all around.

Here was a people who owed everything to their tiny patches of the earth. Their claim to these was validated by the generations who had lived and died before them, toiled and been buried in the same soil. This was the life of the burned girl, of Sangala, Flemings and Lysard Moyo – and

I sensed in all of them an instinctual rightfulness to their place in the world.

I knew no such feeling growing up in a Western metropolis, remote from nature, a stranger among so many others. I was an 'anywhere' person: I might relocate to any other large city, and my life would be essentially the same. In Malaŵi I could observe – from a distance – what it meant to belong somewhere.

To discover my connection with people and places, I had – like Banda – to turn to stories from the past, Classics, history, literature. For me, it was poets like Thomas and Eliot that most explicitly answered this need, and I sensed that many Malaŵian writers pursued the same end: salvaging myths, explaining ancient reflexes, re-inventing ancestral certitudes for our unguided present. The alternative was the life of mental nomadism spreading throughout the West – easy because unattached, but unsettled and unconsoled.

XXXIX

OLD FIELDS, NEW CORN

Remoteness characterised Banda's final years. He was shuttled from palace to palace by Rolls-Royce and helicopter. As he advanced in decrepitude, his engagement with government dwindled, and his trips abroad grew longer. In London he might spend months in a suite at Claridge's Hotel. There, in 1985, he invited the Queen and Margaret Thatcher to a formal banquet to reciprocate his reception at Windsor. Lake fish was flown in specially by Air Malaŵi and paired with vintage Meursault. White ties and sashes, tiaras and decorations shimmered on sergeants-at-arms and ladies-in-waiting.

Banda always had a dangerous tendency to pomposity and long-windedness. Now he stood before his guests, mumbling solemnly, recounting platitudes and unamusing anecdotes that were met with the saccharine smiles of diplomacy. Auden, as so often, had a phrase for it: here was the elderly rubbish that dictators talk to an apathetic grave.

After this, the assembled dignitaries were treated to excerpts from the Malaŵi Civil Service's recent staff revue, which bore the title *Zikomo, Kamuzu!* – 'Thank you, Kamuzu!' Banda's triumphal role in a number of episodes from Malaŵian history was acted out, and, at the end, the chorus summed up with a punchy peroration: 'All improvements in standards of living are attributable to Kamuzu and to Kamuzu alone!'

Sycophancy had long prevailed at Banda's court, the natural corollary of the high-handed approach he took from the start. Talent was driven out soon after independence, in fear of the usurpation to which so many of his fellow African presidents succumbed. His MPs were treated like schoolboys, his ministers like house prefects, all adherent to a strict dress code, with the latter expected to present themselves in morning tails and kid gloves. 'I am pleased to note that the standard of debate is much improved this year,' Banda observed drily at one closing of parliament. It was like the head master's end-of-term assembly.

Banda began to work only alternate mornings, during which time documents would be waved before him for his signature by a coterie of ministers jostling for attention. In the afternoons, he would walk in the grounds of whichever palace he was occupying, read his works of history and nap. Malaŵi's government became geriatric just as its people were drifting into demographic catastrophe and the HIV pandemic. The country became mired in autocracy, dysfunctionality and injustice, albeit without the degree of horror which characterised politics elsewhere on the continent. Death tolls in nearby countries, often running into the hundreds of thousands, were on a different scale. But that does not exculpate: in Malaŵi, people *were* killed, beaten, imprisoned, terrorised.

> When you've never lived under
> a despot admit it, his minions never
> made you dance in the flaming heat
> nor forced you to offer your last cow,
> goat, sheep, chicken, egg or coin.
> When you've never lived under

> the despot's minions confess, you will
> never feel the hit squads that bumped off
> the political rebels they fashioned
> for their president for life, forever
> poisoning the nation.
> When you've never truly lived under
> a despot and his ferocious dogsbodies
> acknowledge, otherwise you'll never
> spot the larger plot.

Mapanje's challenge in 'When You've Never Lived Under a Despot' is a fair one, and I am conscious of my own good fortune. But you don't need the example of Banda to know that the past is full of cruelty, injustice, waste and failure – and there are other lessons that can be learnt from his story.

I have heard the same phrase echoed by many Malaŵians, even his would-be detractors: 'Dr Banda – he *cared*.'

His ideals might have been eclectic, sometimes abhorrent, mostly unfulfilled, but they were sincere. The one that interests me is his desire to protect, celebrate and bring together the two cultures he loved, the African and European. Was anything achieved in this? Can Banda take the credit? Did he just embarrass both the local culture and the one he imported? Readers can judge for themselves.

Pa gule, fumbi ndiwe mwini, Kamuzu. The dust is yours, they say in Malaŵi, referring to the cloud kicked up in the arena by the stamping feet of the *gule* dancer. Show yourself, dance your dance, face the music, for good or ill – that is how I would interpret this characteristically gnomic Chewa proverb, which seems apt for one whose legacy is so ambiguous. Banda's record sometimes reads like a case study in coincidence and unintended consequences. He was 'the tyrant who at a swish of his fly-whisk mowed people into dust', wrote the poet Lupenga Mphande, 'unaware that even dust will rise in the wind and soar to the sky'.

Pentheus, in Dr Highbrow's play, was acted by Mtendere who, with his Homeric dictionary in one hand, a saxophone in the other, was as eccentric a graduate of Kamuzu Academy as Banda could have hoped for. Torn between the arts and the sciences, he won a full scholarship to the country's medical school. At the time of writing, he has just completed his degree and hopes one day to join Malaŵi's tiny body of neurosurgeons. Still stirred by memories of the *Odyssey*, he is composing an epic poem about Kamuzu Banda's wanderings and the reading of Greek in remote places.

Mtendere's contemporary, Matalina, was an orphan and government scholar who excelled in Latin grammar and prose composition. On leaving the academy, she applied these skills to the study of Mandarin Chinese and recently completed a long scholarship in a remote province of the People's Republic.

And then there is Ekari, who came to the academy from a remote village in the south, the son of an occasional bricklayer who earns considerably less than a dollar a day, if he has work. Ekari was unusual in taking both Latin and Greek to A level and applied twice to the University of Cambridge, which showed little interest in the peculiarity of his circumstances. When pursued between applications by Dr Highbrow, an admissions officer there wondered whether, as an African, Ekari wouldn't be better off studying something more useful. And so Ekari was returned to his village and its life of illiteracy and subsistence farming for two more years. Dr Highbrow, however, continued to make representations on his behalf with various academic contacts. To his surprise, he one day received a message from a small institution in Rome: the Accademia Vivarium Novum.

The AVN ploughs a lonely furrow promoting spoken Latin and Greek in conditions that approximate the monastic. Almost nobody, it should be emphasised, at Oxford, Cambridge or elsewhere, has been able to *speak* Latin or Greek for a very long time. At AVN, the approach is total immersion, and students of all ages enrol for at least a year. They live together on a campus beyond the suburbs of Rome and communicate only in Latin and Greek. Modern languages are forbidden, with no exception made even for the estate handyman and driver. When the staff lost my suitcase, I was both frustrated and amused that the plan for its recovery was explained to me only in Latin.

Pauperiores ante ceteros is one of AVN's guiding principles. 'The poorer students come before the rest.' There was an interview via a borrowed cell-phone, which Dr Highbrow had to convey 200 miles to Ekari's village. Soon after, AVN offered a full scholarship, including board and lodging, for two years. Dr Highbrow and I had only to find him his air fare, visa, warm clothes, pocket money and a passport – the first anyone in his family had possessed.

I pressed UK friends for funds, while Dr Highbrow rose to the occasion in Malaŵi, dispatching agents up and down the country to obtain the documentation. Anyone familiar with bureaucracy in sub-Saharan Africa will understand that this was Sisyphean work. For the visa, Dr Highbrow had to convey Ekari across the border to Zambia, where they were put up by Catholic missionaries in Lusaka during the long period of negotiation with the Italian Embassy. Astonishingly, everything was assembled just in time for the start of term, and Ekari found himself boarding an aircraft for the first time in his life, waved off by Dr Highbrow at Kamuzu International Airport.

The explicit goal of AVN is to foster a community dedicated to the ideals of humanism, as expressed in the highest literature, art and music available to man. The languages are just the point of access to that. 'We are reliving the Renaissance here,' Ekari wrote to me soon after his arrival. 'The goal is to teach not Latin or Greek but *humanitas*. I am very thankful for this opportunity. I will not have another chance to live this life again for it does not exist anywhere else. Speaking Latin is not exactly easy, but I am slowly getting the hang of it.'

I visited him a few months later, my arrival occasioning a flurry of activity as earnest-looking young men dashed around the cloisters calling to each other: '*Vidistine Ekarium?! Vidistine Ekarium?!*'

At last, he ambled towards me, chatting remarkably fluently with two friends. But when we met, we reverted to Malaŵian English, and the comforting reflex of the country's universal formulaic greeting:

'Hello, sir, how are you?'

'I am fine, thank you, Ekari. What about you?'

'I am also fine, thank you.'

'Thank you.'

Even, or especially, when meeting Malaŵians abroad, there is a stirring of kinship merely at the exchange of those formal but warm and familiar words of greeting.

AVN's students seldom leave the campus: they live together, eat together, take classes together, and contact with the outside world is minimal. There is no television, no radio and no music they do not make themselves. In the evenings they sing, in Latin. Mobile phone use is discouraged, and access to one or two computers carefully regulated. Literature is the mainstay of leisure time, and the students read voraciously. Within one year, Ekari had read more Latin than I had done throughout my four as an undergraduate.

It is a dirty secret of Classics teaching in the UK that almost nobody even aspires to *speak* Latin or Greek. After two years, Ekari was fairly fluent in both. He could also read any Greek or Roman author without recourse to the dictionaries, grammars and parallel translations on which Oxbridge classicists are wholly dependent. Early on, he rendered his CV and a personal statement into Latin and Greek. Soon he was writing essays in Latin and, in his second year, a dissertation on the role of free will and fate in the philosophy of Seneca.

Most remarkable was how natural a figure Ekari cut in that extraordinary scene. AVN's students come from across Europe, Asia and the Americas, and most have a curious tale to tell. Elsewhere, Ekari might have stuck out; here he could blend in. Despite its unapologetically Eurocentric curriculum, AVN achieved a cultural diversity that would make the rest of Western academe jealous. Only Britain seemed under-represented in the student body.

This diversity was accompanied by neither self-congratulation nor ostentation – it was simply taken for granted. Ekari was not condescended to, feted or exhibited. The students all needed urgently to master the universal language so they could actually communicate. As they lost themselves to this task, the differences between them seemed to evanesce. I wonder if this would have been Ekari's experience at any other school in Europe.

After two years at AVN, Ekari moved to America, where the University of Kentucky offered him a scholarship to pursue postgraduate studies in Classics. He began working on a thesis on the second-century Greek novelist Lucian, whose *True History* is a work of proto-science fiction about impossible journeys to improbable worlds. I understand he has since completed his master's degree, and a doctorate has been mooted. Possibilities widen before him, but perhaps he still thinks of returning to teach in Malaŵi, where Banda's classical experiment may be yet to play itself out.

Latin and Greek in Africa – what could be more pointless? But cost–benefit analysis can feel petty in Malaŵi, and other values often confound the prejudices of profit and loss. Where the presence of the ancestors is still keenly felt, the modern instinct to jettison the past is weakened. Communication between living and dead is real and important here: that is the lesson of *gule*, of the ancient myths of the Chewa, of the poets who have worked to preserve them. It applies no less to Greece and Rome, Homer and Vergil: they can all speak to us differently after their contact with Africa, as Ekari's example shows. He will probably disagree profoundly with much of this book. But he – better than anyone else – must know how the past can nourish our present, if we attend to it.

XL

APOCOLOCYNTOSIS

The example of Hastings Kamuzu Banda is heavy with bathos. He was once hailed as the Lion of Malaŵi, Chief of Chiefs, Founder and Father of the Nation. According to some, he was even Kachirambe reborn – a hero from ancient legend who had slain a terrible 'pumpkin monster' that once ravaged the land and, in later reworkings of the story, became a symbol of colonialism. But at his end Banda fell far from this godlike status: in his final years he was denounced as a criminal, reviled as a tyrant, disdained as a silly old man, whose follies had mired his people in backwardness.

The flawed hero has a long history in Malaŵi, as does the theme of reconciliation. M'bona was the mythical sorcerer who aroused mistrust because he used his powers for both good and ill. When a catastrophic drought befell the land, he was charged with witchcraft and beheaded.

'M'bona wails to be appeased,' wrote Steve Chimombo in his dramatisation of the story. 'The only salvation is to follow the sacred ordinances. The only course is for the Nyau to perform the proper funeral rites of a great man.' The people heed this warning, and, as soon as M'bona's body is honoured with burial, his spirit proves generous. The spilt blood is magically transformed into a torrent of water, rivers replenish the dead land, and rain begins to fall.

After a little contention, Banda was also laid to rest with due ceremony. The new regime was otherwise keen to vilify his memory, but acquiesced as he was laid into a gold coffin, along with Homburg, fly-whisk and cane. A gun carriage conveyed his body to the grave, past mourners numbered in hundreds of thousands. A military band marched with the bier, playing the eclectic soundtrack of his life: hymns of Scotland, America and Africa interspersed with British pomp inherited through the King's African Rifles. 'Auld Lang Syne' and 'Bringing in the Sheaves'. The low brass of the Beethoven funeral march. 'Nearer, My God, to Thee'.

Some chiefs, especially from the Chewa heartlands, hired buses to convey their people to the capital for the occasion. Sangala was present with his father, but they were far at the back of the crowd. Near them, though, cavorted one or two Nyau dancers, the lion and the elephant, there to facilitate the great chief's transition to 'the village on the other side'.

There is a story in Homer which echoes that of M'bona. Odysseus's companion, Elpenor, has an unheroic end: drunk on the eve of departure from Circe's enchanted island, he stumbles from the roof where he has been sleeping, falls and breaks his neck. When Odysseus later visits the Underworld, Elpenor begs him to return and bury his body with the rites he is due. Only then can he properly join the dead and be no longer a burden to the living, he explains. Undistinguished though his death might have been, he requires honour and a grave, so that after-comers may remember and learn from him. Odysseus and his comrades duly sail back to bury Elpenor. They erect a cairn and set over it the oar with which he once rowed beside them.

I thought of these stories again when I revisited Malaŵi a few years ago. Dr Highbrow had left some months previously, following a similarly inglorious downfall. He had, as the Malaŵian idiom puts it, 'mistaken his job'. Paperwork and administration were not among his strengths, and that summer the pupils discovered, on opening the Greek GCSE exam, that they had been taught the wrong texts for the previous two years. Dr Highbrow, who had misread the syllabus, confessed everything to the exam board. They were persuaded to adjust the marks accordingly, and no pressure was brought to bear on him to resign. Nonetheless, he was too embarrassed to continue, and offered his notice.

He had gone back at last to the UK, leaving his immense library in storage in the far north of Malaŵi. It was his most valued possession, and I suppose he wanted thereby to bind himself to the country and compel his own return one day. For Sangala and his other friends, however, he now felt very far away. Twice a day from Kasungu District you could observe a plane flying north out of Malaŵi, on its way to Addis or Nairobi. But in the context of village life, where just getting to the nearest town could be an insuperable challenge, the sight of those strange machines hurtling through the sky served only to emphasise the unimaginable remoteness of the world to which they flew. From the perspective of Malaŵi, Dr Highbrow had gone.

I was back in the country for other reasons, but the trip felt different without him. Still, I visited Kasungu District and happily coincided with Sangala's promotion in seniority as a chief. He asked me to attend the ceremony at a nearby village, explaining that there would be *gule*, and one dance in particular he wanted me to see.

It was a remote but orderly place, with one or two houses that were even roofed with tin and paned with glass. A large but subdued crowd was present, gathered around an open shelter, which stood not far from the village's own small church. Half a dozen local chiefs were sat in a circle under its shade, old men in whom I recognised the upright bearing of Banda-era dignitaries, all clean-shaven and carefully dressed, albeit in well-worn suits and blazers. Their features were defined with age and experience, and a couple had brilliant white hair. They received me courteously and with impeccable English, bidding me to a chair behind them.

Sangala and his wife knelt in the middle on the floor. Someone then draped squares of fabric over their bowed heads, and the chiefs began to address them. One by one they intoned ancient formulas of good government, warnings and imprecations about how and how not to guide one's people. The fabric was to conceal the identities of the speakers, for the wisdom was to come not from any living individuals but from the ancestors themselves, making use of mortal tongues. They spoke in quick succession and from memory, so the sound that arose was almost like chant. I could understand none of it, but I heard 'Chasama', the name of Sangala's village being intoned again and again. When they had finished, Sangala's head was uncovered, and this name 'Chasama' was now used to address him. He was no longer Sangala: by these rites his name had changed, and he had become one with the place where he would now preside.

Then the *gule* dancers appeared to dignify and consecrate the occasion, leading Sangala off the floor and onto a plastic chair set beside the other chiefs'. We settled down to watch the performance.

'But where are these Nyau from?' I asked. I wanted to know if the dancers were from these chiefs' villages, or from Sangala's own.

'They have come from the grave to dance for us!' Sangala replied, consistent with his previous answers.

'But where do they live normally?' I tried again.

'Oh!' he answered. 'Over there!' And Sangala pointed yonder to a dark clump of trees at the end of a trail through the long grass. Such a clump almost always marked a graveyard, for only in these are the trees preserved rather than felled for firewood. I could make out tombstones set among massive primeval roots that upturned and burst open the soil.

'You see the *gule* graves?' he pointed. Yes, some of the markers were large and ominous in shape. One I could see was a giant concrete rabbit, but the others were also meant to be animal forms.

'Those are the *gule* they dance!' explained Sangala, ambiguously. 'Ah, now you see – this one is Dr Highbrow!'

And indeed, there he was: out of the bushes stomped his large clumsy frame, red-faced, bespectacled, puffing on a straw cigar and brandishing a book. He moved ponderously at first, then broke into a gay, light-footed jig, while behind him trailed red and purple tatters that aped an Oxford DPhil gown. Suddenly he tripped on a log and stumbled exaggeratedly to the ground. The crowd laughed, then cheered as he leapt to his feet, brushed himself off and bowed warmly while skitting round the arena, doffing a mock-up of a tasselled mortar-board hat.

'We call him Mondokwa! You know what it means?'

I did – it was the fresh young maize, eaten raw as a delicacy before it is fully ripe. It is delicious, with a satisfying chewy consistency and a sweet, buttery flavour.

'But why Mondokwa?' I asked.

'Mondokwa is the sweetest maize,' Sangala explained. 'It is the best – but it is finished too soon!' And he gestured expansively to the tumid cobs and burgeoning foliage all around us.

It was a strange mix of apotheosis and incarnation. Dr Highbrow joined the great pantheon of *gule*, with Sangala's forebears, manifold chiefs, Dr Banda himself and all the rest of the ancestors. Yet at the same time their departed spirits were made flesh before us, here and now. They might have looked demonic but were animated by the kindly ghosts of our past, here to guide and protect us.

Now all the village was dancing with the *gule* in rings: men and women, chiefs and yeomen, the living, the dead, and even, in a few gravid bellies, the unborn. Around all this movement, the world stood still, the sun high in the cloudless sky, the trees unrustled by the windless air. Only a richness of swallows mirrored us by circling silently overhead.

It was a timeless moment, an impossible union of past, present and future. This was the Great Dance. History stood still. Decay and regeneration were briefly halted, as bare feet pounded exultantly on that blood-red, life-giving soil.

EPILOGUE

Malaŵi's heroes can take you by surprise. I did not expect any to be celebrated outside Africa, let alone in London, but in September 2022 Trafalgar Square's famous Fourth Plinth was adorned with two new statues: of John Chilembwe, the Malaŵian Baptist minister who led a short-lived rebellion against British rule in 1915; and his friend, an English missionary called John Chorley.

Their sculptor is Samson Kambalu, already mentioned as the alumnus of Kamuzu Academy, whose autobiography described strange manifestations of *gule wamkulu* in the boys' dormitories when he was a pupil there in the 1980s. Kambalu subsequently made his way to England, where he flourished as a writer and artist and is now a professor of contemporary art at Oxford University.

His work for the Fourth Plinth was chosen at a time of bitter controversy for Britain's statues. In the summer of 2020, following the murder of George Floyd by a white policeman in Minnesota, the Black Lives Matter movement erupted in America and then spilled over into Britain. In the ensuing riots, statues were particularly targeted: Edward Colston's was torn down in Bristol, while, in London, those of Winston Churchill and Mahatma Gandhi were daubed with graffiti: 'racist'.

Previous Fourth Plinth installations had been mostly conceptual, post-modern, ironic: a giant plastic rooster and a dollop of whipped cream were two typical examples. After the statues controversy, this sort of studied frivolity suddenly went out of fashion, with more assertive, political public art apparently called for instead. Chilembwe was plucked from obscurity and vaunted as an African who had defied the British Empire. From the BBC to the *New York Times*, media commentary cast his rebellion as an instance of heroic opposition to colonial oppression, a straightforward fable of good versus evil. However, Chilembwe's story is complicated and highly ambiguous. In fact, it cuts to the core of the vexed debate about Britain's imperial past.

Chilembwe grew up in southern Malaŵi in the 1870s, a period when the region was still at the heart of the vast Indian Ocean slave trade, its peoples predated upon by Arabs, their Islamised African accomplices and marauding tribes of the Zulu diaspora. Indeed, Chilembwe's mother seems to have been a slave, his father her Yao captor.

Like Hastings Kamuzu Banda, Chilembwe received his early education from Scottish missionaries. He then became servant to an Englishman called Joseph Booth, a born-again Christian who wandered five continents evangelising on behalf of the various churches between which he switched allegiance over the course of his life. He was a pacifist, a socialist and an ardent critic of colonialism, claiming to have coined the phrase 'Africa for the Africans'.

Booth was also strongly influenced by the millenarianism espoused by the Watch Tower Society, forerunners of today's Jehovah's Witnesses. Jesus Christ was believed to have returned invisibly to Earth in 1874, and to be biding his time until the Battle of Armageddon, scheduled for 1914. The Last Judgement would fall the following year, whereupon the Day of Wrath would cease with the overthrow of Satan's capitalist and imperialist world order. These ideas originated in America but, by the turn of the twentieth century, had attained small followings in British Africa.

Booth did not flourish in Malaŵi. He irritated other missionaries, establishing his own church in proximity to theirs, then trying to lure their followers with promises of money – possible thanks to funding from generous American donors. Despite this, his workers proved unreliable and stole from him. In 1892, at a moment of crisis and isolation, Chilembwe appeared, offering his services. He became a trusted assistant, interpreter and protégé, and Booth fared better with his help. By 1897, however, he was on his travels again, this time setting off for America and taking Chilembwe with him.

In the southern states, the pair found racial acrimony still smouldering in the long shadows of the Civil War. The Ku Klux Klan was ubiquitous, and association between black and white attracted hostility. Walking together in the street, Booth and Chilembwe were sometimes pelted with stones. Yet they were welcomed, even feted, by black congregations, especially the most radical. Among these, debate flourished about the best response to white oppression, but also about how Black Americans could support the evangelisation of Africa. Booth's endeavours in Malaŵi stirred their interest, and his fundraising efforts were rewarded.

Chilembwe, meanwhile, was making lifelong friends, some of whom offered to sponsor his further education in America. He parted company from Booth, enrolling at the Baptist seminary in Lynchburg, Virginia, from which he graduated as a pastor two years later. Returning to Malaŵi in 1900, he founded the Providence Industrial Mission in his home district of Chiradzulu, with support from Black American patrons, who initially sent missionaries of their own to bolster his efforts. (Booth was also back in the country, but did not stay long, leaving for good in 1902.)

Christianity, Commerce and Civilisation were as central to Chilembwe's mission as to any led by Europeans. His stated goal was to bring to his countrymen 'the quickening and enlightening influence of the Gospel of Christ to lift them from their state of degradation and make them suitable members of the great human family'. Besides building an impressive church, Chilembwe was also developing a plantation where his followers grew cotton and coffee, one of several belonging to a new local elite of educated, land-owning Africans. Among these, Chilembwe enjoyed great distinction on account of his rare experiences abroad, but he had also become an outsider.

His radical ideas – acquired from Booth and in America – put him at odds not only with colonial society, but also with his own 'benighted people', of whom he often wrote with frustration and disdain. As he contemplated marriage, he observed that 'the ordinary African woman in her heathen state is ignorant, uninteresting and unlovable'.

'I almost despair', he went on, 'when I think of her ignorance, her utter lack of ambition.' His own wife, Ida, seems to have been of mixed Portuguese and African ancestry. She worked with him at the mission, taking charge of a progressive programme of female education.

The Chilembwes had at least three children and enjoyed a little prosperity as they settled into the sort of bourgeois existence that was becoming possible in the country. Again like Banda, Chilembwe was obsessed with his attire as a mark of status, insisting on high standards of dress and deportment from all around him. In one photograph, he sits at the edge of the forest in a check suit and bow tie, a boater on the ground before him. His wife wears a floor-length Victorian gown, complete with gigot sleeves and ruff. You sense that Chilembwe was often over-dressed, in a way that Europeans would have liked to notice with a sneer.

The white population was never large and only about 800 in 1914, out of a total population of 1.25 million. Most Europeans were missionaries and administrators, but there was a small number of settlers who had laid claim to some of the best land, often dishonestly. Nonetheless, this constituted only a small proportion of the whole, and it was shortage of manpower rather than of territory that constrained the colonial economy.

Around this time, the Portuguese in Mozambique instituted a system of forced labour, which – in conjunction with a vicious and arbitrary penal system – impelled tens of thousands to cross the border into British territory. 'This place is wonderful' ran the refrain of a popular song from the period, which was still being sung in the 1980s, in memory of conditions under British rule. Indeed, these economic migrants continued to 'vote with their feet' long after Chilembwe's rebellion.

Nevertheless, many estates were run rapaciously, and conditions on some were appalling, especially for the immigrant groups who made up most of their labour force. In the system known as *thangata*, they were offered tenancy in exchange for work, but the terms could be twisted, and the rules favoured the landowners. Corporal punishment was commonly administered, and labourers might face eviction if they did not comply with employers' demands.

The nearest estate to Chilembwe's mission was Magomero, consisting of 260 square miles that had been bought, bullied or wangled from local chiefs by descendants of David Livingstone, capitalising on their association with the revered explorer. Magomero was the largest estate in the country and had a particular reputation for brutality. Its manager, William Jervis Livingstone, eyed Chilembwe with suspicion from the start, and the two began a feud that lasted many years. Their disagreements were variously petty and profound: there was a bitter argument about a bell, but Chilembwe also used his ministry to denounce conditions under Livingstone's management. Relations eventually got so bad that Chilembwe was banned from evangelising at

Magomero, and the satellite churches and schools he had supported there were demolished. In response, he intensified his rhetoric, preaching avoidance of taxes and identifying Livingstone as the Antichrist.

Chilembwe was floundering. He had always divided opinion within the white community, though some Europeans had initially been supportive of his efforts. Now he became the focus of hostility, but, even so, his remonstrations against colonial society were grudgingly tolerated until 1914, when the Germans invaded Malaŵi from their vast colony to the north. Chilembwe wrote a letter to the *Central African Times* denouncing the war effort, whereupon the government turned decisively against him. His health had deteriorated, his business ventures were struggling, and he had fallen into debt. It was also the year prophesied for Apocalypse. Learning of an official plan to deport him, Chilembwe incited his congregation to rebellion, seemingly aware that this was a reckless, even futile course of action.

His followers were members of his congregation, which was drawn mostly from the misused population of immigrant workers on the estates. He also had a handful of lieutenants who were affluent, educated locals like himself. The total number of rebels is difficult to estimate, but probably around a few hundred: membership of Chilembwe's mission was reported as 900 in 1912, and a list of 175 accomplices was discovered at his church by government forces after the rebellion.

On the night of 23 January 1915, Chilembwe ordered three attacks: on Livingstone's house at Magomero, on a second neighbouring estate and on the offices of the African Lakes Company in Blantyre, where firearms were believed to be stored. From the last of these, Chilembwe's men were quickly repulsed, but the attacks on the estates fared better.

At Magomero, Livingstone was playing with his baby while his wife took her evening bath. The rebels broke inside the house and, for a while, chased him from room to room as he tried to fend them off with an unloaded rifle. Eventually one struck him with an axe, but he managed to stagger into his wife's bedroom and she locked the door. It was soon smashed in, whereupon Livingstone was pinned down and decapitated in front of her and the children. One of his colleagues was also stabbed to death, as were another manager and his Malaŵian servant at the second estate attacked by the rebels. In accordance with Chilembwe's instructions, women and children were taken prisoner but left unharmed.

Chilembwe did not participate in any of these actions, but, the next day, he led a church service beneath Livingstone's severed head, which had been set on a pole. He then retired to pray while a small skirmish took place with government forces, but the rebellion was petering out. A final attack was made on a nearby Catholic mission, where the rebels found the place already evacuated, apart from one sick child and a lone missionary who had stayed behind to look after her. They tried to spear him to death, but he later recovered from his wounds.

Government forces consisted of a civilian militia, a handful of British soldiers and Malaŵian askaris, most of whom were away in the far north, fighting the Germans. Despite this, the few who were at hand easily restored order within a few days. As resistance died out, they began rounding up suspects, often indiscriminately. Several tribes joined the mopping-up operation, some taking advantage of the chaos to settle scores with old enemies. In the aftermath, thirty-six rebels were executed and 300 imprisoned. Chilembwe's church was dynamited, numerous huts were burned, and a fine of four shillings imposed on every man, woman and child as a lesson in collective responsibility. It was a ruthless demonstration of colonial power, but, beyond these reprisals, Chilembwe's rebellion had little immediate impact. A commission of enquiry found fault with the management of the Magomero estate and proposed reform of the *thangata* system. For the most part, life then went on as before.

Chilembwe himself had fled into the forests of Mozambique, where he was hunted down and shot dead by three Malaŵian soldiers. His body was carried back and consigned to an unmarked grave. Before he died, he had written to the Germans, proposing an alliance, though his letter did not reach them in time. It was an unedifying gesture: less than ten years before, Germany had crushed a protracted rebellion in Tanzania with the deaths of perhaps as many as 300,000 people. 'Maji Maji' was a massive revolt that united disparate tribes against a universally detested regime.

Chilembwe's rising was nothing of the sort: despite ten years of fomenting unrest with his sermonising, there was no widespread discontent in colonial Malaŵi at that time. The British were not only tolerated; for many years they enjoyed considerable loyalty from the local population, for whom the extirpation of slavery was a recent memory. Indeed, as word of the rising spread, many chiefs eagerly proclaimed their support for the government.

The most striking thing about Chilembwe is precisely his exceptionalism. Far ahead of his time, he aroused only limited enthusiasm because his perception of injustice was not widely shared. Even his wife Ida expressed bewilderment at her husband's animosity towards the white population. Chilembwe's vision was original: according to his biographer, George Shepperson, other rebellions in colonial Africa had aimed at restoring the fortunes of defeated tribes, whereas Chilembwe's 'looked to the future, not to the past'.

However, the significance of his rebellion was not apparent for some time. Chilembwe was remembered for his courage and defiance, but his example was not otherwise followed. In particular, violent means were disavowed by most of the men and women who worked conscientiously towards their country's independence. When this was achieved in 1964, one of Chilembwe's children – who had been sponsored and educated by the colonial government after the rebellion – was still alive to see it.

In the post-colonial period, sanguinary heroes were more in demand but, even then, Kamuzu Banda tended to be faint with his praise. With a degree of reticence, he commended Chilembwe's intentions, while also disparaging the impracticality of his plan. In 1965, the half centenary of the rebellion was commemorated with a postage stamp. Only in the 1990s, after Banda's downfall, did Chilembwe Day become a national holiday in Malaŵi, as the country's new rulers looked for ways to supplant the cult of the old regime.

It would be easy to dismiss Chilembwe as a figure of well-deserved obscurity, whose final achievement was a crazed, ineffectual act of murderous destruction. And yet there is a poignancy to his story. 'We will all die by the heavy blow of the whiteman's army,' he is reported to have said on the eve of the rebellion. 'The whitemen will think, after we are dead, that the treatment they are treating our people is bad, and they might change to the better for our people.' In these words, there is dignity of purpose as well as real foresight by which it is difficult not to be moved.

This book has insisted we listen for the communication of the dead and, in Kambalu's statues, Chilembwe has achieved a potent, unexpected afterlife. Trafalgar Square is

London's pre-eminent symbol of imperial glory, yet there he stands, face to face with those full-blooded sons of empire, Nelson, Havelock and Napier. It is an arrangement that echoes London's other conciliatory statue pairings, from Cromwell and Charles I to Churchill and Gandhi. History is complicated, they all insist; there are two sides to every story.

As for John Chorley, whose statue shares the plinth, not much is known except that he was Chilembwe's friend. Chorley is cast much smaller, to diminish him and exalt Chilembwe, but it is astonishing that he should be there at all: after the disputes of recent years, it seemed inconceivable that a statue of a white missionary to Africa might be erected anywhere in twenty-first-century Britain. But rancour and recrimination are conspicuously absent from Kambalu's work. Whatever else they may express, his statues urge us to acknowledge missionaries like Chorley, who gave so much to end slavery and foster peace and education in Malaŵi. What would Chilembwe's story have been without them? Might he have followed his father's occupation as a slaver?

Kambalu has portrayed Chilembwe and Chorley both wearing hats, claiming this was illegal for Africans in colonial Malaŵi. This is incorrect and mistakes the character of racism in British Africa, which was seldom enshrined in petty legislation, as in segregated America or under apartheid. It was subtler, more insidious, but perhaps no less poisonous for that.

Hats were certainly a contentious issue, and commissioners at the official enquiry into the rebellion were perplexed that Malaŵian witnesses kept raising the subject. Joseph Bismarck, a wealthy black landowner, played no part in the rebellion and condemned its violence before the commission. However, he took advantage of this platform to articulate the injustices he felt had provoked the rebels. It is a moving account, as he narrates how painfully the insults of Europeans were experienced by his countrymen.

Hats mattered, Bismarck observed, because they were a symbol of 'civilisation'. He often wore a hat, but was expected to remove it in the presence of a white man. Why was this courtesy so seldom reciprocated? And for not removing his hat, Bismarck described how he had been abused with racist slurs and threatened with violence. On one occasion, an Italian planter called him a baboon, and worse.

'I am not a baboon,' Bismarck replied with dignity. 'I am a living being like yourself.'

The planter then pulled a gun.

'Shoot me,' was Bismarck's response.

The commissioners pointed out that Africans had recourse to law if they were mistreated in this way, but clearly it did not work in practice, and, for Bismarck, it wasn't really the point. Educated Malaŵians like himself admired the British, but, when they tried to emulate them, their efforts were spat back in their faces.

The veteran Scots missionary Alexander Hetherwick pointedly averred that black and white should both raise their hats 'because it shows two gentlemen have met and not just one'. But this view was not shared by everyone; nastiness and belittling were widespread. Bismarck and Chilembwe were derided for being 'jumped up' and 'aping their betters'. 'A pitiable travesty' was one newspaper's comment on Chilembwe's missionary efforts. Such expressions of contempt could clearly be deeply wounding, perhaps even more so because the British were respected.

After the rebellion, Chilembwe's house was looted, his possessions dispersed. In a curious historical twist, one of the books in his collection, a biography of David

Livingstone, recently resurfaced in a Malaŵian archive. On the front page, beside his signature, Chilembwe also inscribed some lines of Longfellow:

> Lives of great men all remind us
> We can make our lives sublime,
> And, departing, leave behind us
> Footprints in the sands of time

Poor Chilembwe: a more problematic 'great man' can scarcely be imagined, yet our sententious age needs urgently to be reminded that heroes invariably have their flaws. In atonement for his own, perhaps Chilembwe can teach us to judge our ancestors more generously and to learn from statues, instead of toppling them. First, though, his ghost must be laid to rest. The funeral is overdue, so let it be ungrudging. The Fourth Plinth can be his cenotaph, and a place for us all to make peace with our past.

ACKNOWLEDGEMENTS

My thanks are due first to my editor Michael Holman and my agent Kelly Falconer, not only for their numerous and important improvements to *Goodbye, Dr Banda* but, above all, for their energy and determination to see it published.

I am likewise indebted to Hugh Andrew, Edward Crossan, Jan Rutherford and the rest of the team at Polygon for their hard work and dedication throughout the long process of this book's production.

I received invaluable comments on various iterations of the text from a wide array of sources. They all helped me to improve the book, which is consequently stronger in argument, style, and historical literacy. I would like to acknowledge my debt to Tony Daniels, Jacob Willer, Leon Marshall, Lalya Lloyd, Statten Roeg, Katie Prescott, Jason Pedicone, Bijan Omrani, Gabriella Stubbs, David Stuart-Mogg, John Lwanda, Louis Nthenda, Nigel Biggar and the late Roger Scruton. For any outstanding defects I am wholly responsible.

The last few years were sad ones for writers on Malaŵian affairs, the deaths of several of the most eminent having all occurred in a short span of time. I deeply regret that I was unable to make the acquaintance of so many that have now passed away (especially Owen Kalinga, John McCracken and George Shepperson), but others I had the great privilege to meet or correspond with before they died.

The passing of D.D. Phiri leaves an unfillable gap in the field of Malaŵian history, and I count myself very lucky that I was able to talk to him about my book. The memory of our one meeting in Blantyre the year before he died remains vivid, as much for his warmth and marvellous eccentricity as for his vast learning.

Less focussed on Malaŵi specifically, but nevertheless endowed with an extraordinary knowledge of the region were Donal Lowry and Tom Stacey. I remember both with affection and gratitude for the generosity with which they shared their wealth of knowledge and experience, and for their personal encouragement with my book. They are deeply missed.

More happily, this project has been the occasion to make contact with several Malaŵian writers whose work I admire. I am particularly grateful to Felix Mnthali for permitting me to reproduce his poems. His support has meant a great deal to me, and I hope that my book can serve as a tribute to and reminder of his remarkable literary achievement, which is too little known beyond Africa. Similarly, I would like to express my thanks to the family of Landeg White for permission to quote his poetry, and to Moira Chimombo for permission to quote that of her late husband Steve. Moira has also been very kind in sharing her memories of the extraordinary literary world they together inhabited.

Above all, though, this book could never have been written without the openness and generosity of countless Malaŵians who – in such a variety of ways – granted me some access to their lives. I have in mind everything from brief, anonymous interactions to ongoing friendships that can be traced to my earliest acquaintance with the country. It would be impossible to enumerate all of these, but I would like to express particular gratitude to Mabel Banda, Mike Banda, Tamali Banda, Annie Chidali, Chikondi Chidzanja, Davis Chikoti, James and Grace Chisale, Hawkins Gondwe, Peter and Jacqueline Minjale, John Nkhata and his family, Peter and Samson Phiri. I am also indebted to the Burgess and Pyman families and to Frans and Ardine Zoetmulder for both their hospitality and their readiness to talk about their long experiences of Malaŵi.

Finally, I am exceedingly grateful to Mama Cecilia Kadzamira and her wider family for their kindness and generosity in sharing their memories. I appreciate that aspects of this book might disappoint them, but I hope they will nevertheless recognise the sympathy and good faith with which I have written about the extraordinary Dr Banda.

The author and publisher would like to thank the following authors, publishers and estates who have generously given permission to reproduce the extracts from the following poems:

'East Coker' by T.S. Eliot from *The Four Quartets* (Faber, 1944) by permission of Faber and Faber; 'Skipping Without Rope', 'Before Chilembwe Tree', 'When You've Never Lived Under a Despot' by Jack Mapanje from *The Last of the Sweet Bananas: New & Selected Poems* (Bloodaxe Books, 2004) by permission of the publisher; 'Neocolonialism', 'Palaces in the Jungle' and 'December seventh, 'Seventy-six' by Felix Mnthali by permission of the author; 'A Peasant' by R.S. Thomas from *Selected Poems 1946–1968* (Bloodaxe Books, 1986) by permission of the publisher; 'In the Village' by Landeg White, from *Mau* (Hetherwick Press, 1971) by permission of the trustees of Landeg White's literary estate.

Every effort has been made to trace copyright holders of the quotes in this book. The author and publisher apologise if any material has been included without appropriate acknowledgement and would be glad to receive any information on authors and their estates we have not been able to trace.